Urodynamics Made Easy

Third Edition

Christopher R Chapple BSc MBBS MD FRCS(Urol) FEBU

Consultant Urological Surgeon, Sheffield Teaching Hospitals, Royal Hallamshire
Hospital, Sheffield, UK;
Professor of Urology, Sheffield Hallam University, Sheffield

Scott A MacDiarmid MD

Director, Alliance Urology Specialists, Bladder Control and Pelvic Pain Center, North
Carolina, USA;
Clinical Faculty, Department of Urology, Wake Forest University, Winston-Salem,
North Carolina, USA

Anand Patel MB ChB MRCS

Urology Research Fellow, Sheffield Teaching Hospitals, Royal Hallamshire Hospital,
Sheffield, UK

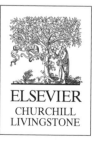

ELSEVIER
CHURCHILL
LIVINGSTONE

Edinburgh   London   New York   Oxford   Philadelphia   St Louis   Sydney   Toronto   2009

ELSEVIER
CHURCHILL
LIVINGSTONE

ISBN: 978-0-443-06886-7

British Library Cataloguing in Publication Data
A catalogue record for this book is available from the British Library

Library of Congress Cataloging in Publication Data
A catalog record for this book is available from the Library of Congress

Notice
Knowledge and best practice in this field are constantly changing. As new
research and experience broaden our knowledge, changes in practice,
treatment and drug therapy may become necessary or appropriate. Readers
are advised to check the most current information provided (i) on
procedures featured or (ii) by the manufacturer of each product to be
administered, to verify the recommended dose or formula, the method and
duration of administration, and contraindications. It is the responsibility of
the practitioner, relying on their own experience and knowledge of the
patient, to make diagnoses, to determine dosages and the best treatment for
each individual patient, and to take all appropriate safety precautions. To
the fullest extent of the law, neither the Publisher nor the Authors assume
any liability for any injury and/or damage to persons or property arising
out of or related to any use of the material contained in this book.

The Publisher

Printed in Spain

Contents

Preface

This book aims to dispel the image that urodynamics is a complex subject. Urodynamics is not an esoteric subject of limited applicability and requiring complex equipment that is best confined to the 'ivory towers'. The basic principles of urodynamics are simple and in most cases complex investigation is unnecessary.

Factors that have fostered the popular erroneous image that urodynamics is complex are:

- First, the application of theoretical physics to the subject – although producing useful models on which to base further research, this is of limited use to the practising clinician. It is, however, useful to consider the urinary tract as a series of conduits within which urine movement is dictated by the pressures acting upon them and their resistance to flow, with specific sphincteric mechanisms acting as zones of variable resistance.

- Second, the use of jargon terms that have tended to complicate and obscure otherwise logical and straightforward concepts. To clarify this, the official terminology relating to urodynamics (presented in the format specified by the International Continence Society) is reviewed in this book.

This guide outlines the principles and practice of urodynamics in the routine clinical management of patients. Although the 'bladder is an unreliable witness' and is associated with a variety of non-specific symptoms, improvements in urodynamic techniques and electronic equipment over the past 20 years have allowed the widespread use of objective investigations to clarify these symptoms.

Urodynamics is the study of pressure and flow relationships during the storage and transport of urine within the urinary tract. In routine practice most urodynamic investigations are focused on the lower urinary tract to:

- investigate bladder filling and voiding function
- accurately define bladder storage disorders and
- assess the severity of voiding dysfunction.

Upper tract urodynamics is usually carried out in specialist units.

The first edition of this book was compiled with Tim Christmas who due to other commitments has been unable to participate in the authorship of future editions. I was then delighted to work with Scott MacDiarmid, a longstanding friend and colleague working in the USA. More recently my research fellow Anand Patel has joined the team. Together we have fully updated and further expanded on the scope of the book, in particular, adding in appendices showing a schemata for performing a pressure/flow study, a glossary of normal urodynamic values and annotated example traces.

CRC, May 2008

Foreword

This third edition of *Urodynamics Made Easy* is a tribute to the sustained vision of the authors and a unique opportunity for them to continue to share their longstanding experience with urodynamic testing. Urodynamics is a fascinating discipline in full expansion, which has benefited recently from remarkable technical and scientific advances.

Adding to the prior versions, this edition offers a fresh look at the latest refinements in equipment. Current urodynamic consoles have become ergonomic, offer fast processing, are equipped with digital imaging and large memories, and deliver various physician-friendly, well-annotated, and colourful interpretation reports.

The 10 chapters cover a large range of topics including urinary symptoms and current term definitions endorsed by the International Continence Society, urodynamic techniques, and diagnostic findings related to incontinence, obstruction, sensory disorders, neurogenic bladder, and paediatric urology. The presentation of each chapter is uniform with a concise text and practical, colour-coded tables illustrating and emphasizing key messages regarding typical urodynamic findings. In addition, several didactic tracings are offered in appendix, along with a section on normative values and a short bibliography.

Lessons learned from urodynamics performed in large multicentric trials like the Urinary Incontinence Treatment Network in the US have helped not only in the design of simplified testing protocols for women with stress incontinence, including standardized annotations, but also in reaching new frontiers such as consensus in interpretation guidelines and inter-rater reliability studies across several reviewers (www.uitn.net/documents/UDS_Protocol_020206.pdf). Moreover, there is recognition that a broader teaching and training of urodynamic skills needs to be incorporated in our residency education programs. In this light, the timing of this third edition is ideal, as it represents a great and simple teaching tool that will assist the novice as well as the more experienced practitioner.

Clearly, urodynamic labs and testers should be encouraged to have this edition at their fingertips. Likewise, all those interested in growing their understanding of and expertise in pelvic floor diseases should use this invaluable and practical yet comprehensive resource.

Philippe E Zimmern

Acknowledgements

Our thanks go to the International Continence Society (ICS) for its permission to reproduce figures and definitions from its documents on standardization. We would also like to thank the following specialist nurses (based at the Royal Hallamshire Hospital, Sheffield, UK) for reviewing sections of the manuscript: Sister Carol Fleet, Sister Anne Frost and Sister Rachel Simmons.

The following companies kindly provided information regarding current urodynamic equipment, figures and urodynamic traces for inclusion in this book:

Gaeltec
Dunvegan
Isle of Skye
IV55 8GU
Scotland
www.gaeltec.com

Genesis Medical Limited
7 Trojan Business Centre
Cobbold Road
London
NW10 9ST
UK
www.genmedhealth.com

Laborie Medical Technologies
6415 Northwest Drive
Unit 11, Mississauga
Ontario
L4V 1X1
Canada
www.laborie.com

Medical Measurement Systems (MMS)
P.O. Box 580
7500 AN Enschede
The Netherlands
www.mmsinternational.com

T-Doc Company, LLC
5 Edgemoor Road
Suite 212
Wilmington, DE 19809
USA
www.tdocllc.com

CHAPTER 1

Clinical evaluation of the lower urinary tract

INTRODUCTION

The bladder and the urethra comprise the lower urinary tract and act as a single (vesico-urethral) unit during normal lower urinary tract function. The role of this unit is to:

- adequately store urine (storage)
- efficiently empty urine (voiding).

If the function of this vesico-urethral unit is disturbed then urinary dysfunction along with associated lower urinary tract symptoms (LUTS) may occur. Management of lower urinary tract dysfunction is based on the findings of:

- a focused history and physical examination
- appropriate laboratory studies
- endoscopy and radiography – to provide structural information when clinically indicated
- urodynamic studies – to provide functional information when clinically indicated.

FOCUSED HISTORY AND PHYSICAL EXAMINATION

First and foremost, a focused history establishes a working diagnosis, helps formulate clinical questions and directs subsequent investigations and management. Previously a plethora of overlapping and confusing terms relating to lower urinary tract dysfunction were in usage; however the International Continence Society (ICS) have published terminology reports to standardize the terms used when describing LUTS. Thus, enabling consistent and accurate reporting of symptoms and enabling further investigations and management to be appropriately directed. It is recommended that only standardized terminology is used when describing LUTS.

The ICS have broadly categorized LUTS into three groups (Table 1.1) related to their timing within the bladder (voiding) cycle. The three stages of the bladder cycle are:

Lower urinary tract symptoms		
Storage	**Voiding**	**Post-micturition**
Urgency	Hesitancy	Feeling of incomplete emptying
Increased daytime frequency	Intermittency	Post-micturition dribble
Nocturia	Slow stream	
Urinary incontinence	Splitting or spraying	
Altered bladder sensation	Straining	
	Terminal dribble	

Table 1.1 *Lower urinary tract symptoms.*

1. **Storage** – during which passive filling of the bladder occurs, either naturally from urine produced by the kidneys or artificially during a urodynamic study.
2. **Voiding** – during which the vesico-urethral unit actively expels the bladder contents.
3. **Post-micturition** – immediately after voiding when the bladder returns to storage function.

Specific definitions for lower urinary tract symptoms are listed in the box at the end of this chapter.

The bladder is frequently said to be an 'unreliable witness'. There are a number of reasons why this statement accurately reflects the situation. First, lower urinary tract symptoms are not disease specific and diverse patho-physiologies can produce similar lower urinary tract symptoms. Second, patients express symptoms in different ways and this is influenced both by what they are experiencing and how they interpret the symptoms they are experiencing. Lastly, as clinicians we all take histories differently and interpret the clinical picture based on our own experience and prejudices.

Clearly however, a careful history with emphasis on allocating symptoms to the appropriate stage of the bladder cycle is an important starting point. Failure to store can be due to overactivity of the bladder, underactivity of the bladder with overflow, or weakness of the bladder outlet. Likewise, while voiding symptoms tend to be associated in many people's minds with bladder outlet obstruction, they can of course also occur in the context of poor bladder function.

Having taken a careful history and carried out an appropriate clinical examination; laboratory, endoscopic or radiographic tests should be performed prior to urodynamic assessment as clinically indicated.

URODYNAMIC EVALUATION

Appropriate urodynamic tests can only be interpreted after taking an adequate history, with the formulation of specific clinical questions; since the principal aims of the urodynamic assessment are to answer the clinical questions by evaluating the function of the vesico-urethral unit. Urodynamics is particularly of benefit in objectively identifying *functional* abnormalities of the lower urinary tract such as urinary incontinence and bladder outflow obstruction (BOO). However (particularly with video cystometry) it may also assist in identifying *structural* abnormalities such as a prolapse associated with stress urinary incontinence (SUI), vesico-vaginal fistulae, urethral diverticula, upper tract vesico-ureteric reflux; or in the context of the male patient, it can be useful in demonstrating attenuation of the prostatic urethra in association with prostatic outlet obstruction or confirming the diagnosis of bladder neck obstruction.

The term 'urodynamics' encompasses any investigation of lower urinary tract dysfunction from the simple to the sophisticated, these include:

- Frequency/volume chart (FVC).
- Bladder diary.
- Pad testing.
- Uroflowmetry ± ultrasound residual estimation.
- Pressure/flow studies:
  - cystometry
  - video cystometry
  - ambulatory urodynamics.
- Urethral pressure studies.
- Other studies:
  - intravenous urodynamogram
  - ultrasound cystodynamogram.

The most frequently performed tests are FVC/bladder diaries, uroflowmetry and pressure/flow studies.

Generally the term 'urodynamics' has become synonymous with pressure/flow studies, with most clinicians referring to either cystometry or video cystometry when they use the term "urodynamics".

3

URODYNAMICS IN PRACTICE

Urodynamics:
- can only be interpreted in association with a comprehensive history and examination of the patient, where they are valuable adjuncts in the investigation of patients who have LUTS/lower urinary tract dysfunction
- have become synonymous with pressure/flow studies, with most clinicians referring to either cystometry or video cystometry
- are objective functional tests of bladder and urethral function (and may provide some associated structural information)
- may help indicate the most appropriate therapy.

Indication and interpretation of urodynamics

The information acquired from accurately interpreted and well performed urodynamic studies can be used to:
- diagnose the underlying cause of the lower urinary tract dysfunction
- characterize the lower urinary tract dysfunction
- formulate treatment strategies
- improve therapeutic outcomes
- educate patients regarding their condition.

An experienced clinician with an understanding of urodynamic techniques should carry out the urodynamic study and should interpret the study in the context of the patient's symptoms. As with all practical skills there is a learning curve, with the interpretation becoming easier with increasing experience. The authors believe that the true clinical value or 'art' of urodynamics is in applying the objective findings of a well executed study to the individual patient, taking into consideration subtleties in the history and physical examination that may be clinically important.

LOWER URINARY TRACT SYMPTOM TERMINOLOGY

It is essential to use standardized terminology when discussing lower urinary tract symptoms (LUTS) and the results of urodynamic investigations, to allow accurate exchange and comparison of information for clinical and research purposes. The official terminology suggested by the International Continence Society (ICS) in 2002 is used throughout this book. The ICS terminology for LUTS is summarized below and the terminology for urodynamic parameters are defined in later chapters. Further information regarding terminology can be found on the ICS website (www.icsoffice.org).

TERMINOLOGY: LOWER URINARY TRACT SYMPTOMS

Storage symptoms

- **Increased daytime frequency:** the complaint by the patient who considers that he/she voids too often by day (term is equivalent to pollakisuria used in many countries).
- **Nocturia:** the complaint that the patient has to wake at night one or more times to void.
- **Urgency:** a sudden compelling desire to pass urine which is difficult to defer.
- **Urinary incontinence (UI):** any involuntary leakage of urine.
- **Stress urinary incontinence (SUI):** involuntary leakage on effort or exertion, or on sneezing or coughing.
- **Urge(ncy) urinary incontinence (UUI):** involuntary leakage accompanied by or immediately preceded by *urgency* (urge urinary incontinence is a misnomer since it is urgency that is associated with this incontinence and we therefore believe it should be called 'urgency incontinence', not urge incontinence).
- **Mixed urinary incontinence (MUI):** involuntary leakage associated with urgency and also with exertion, effort, sneezing or coughing (a mixture of urgency urinary incontinence and stress urinary incontinence symptoms).
- **Mixed urinary symptoms:** involuntary leakage associated with exertion, effort, sneezing or coughing; combined with urgency but not urge(ncy) incontinence
- **Enuresis:** any involuntary loss of urine (similar to definition of urinary incontinence).
- **Nocturnal enuresis:** loss of urine occurring during sleep (involuntary symptom, as opposed to 'nocturia' which is a voluntary and 'conscious' symptom).
- **Continuous urinary incontinence:** the complaint of continuous leakage.
- **Other types of urinary incontinence:** may be situational, for example incontinence during sexual intercourse, or giggle incontinence.

Bladder sensations during storage phase

- **Normal bladder sensation:** aware of bladder filling and increasing sensation up to a strong desire to void.
- **Increased bladder sensation:** aware of an early and persistent desire to void.
- **Reduced bladder sensation:** aware of bladder filling but does not feel a definite desire to void.
- **Absent bladder sensation:** no awareness of bladder filling or desire to void.
- **Non-specific bladder sensation:** no specific bladder sensation but may perceive bladder filling as abdominal fullness, or spasticity (these are most frequently seen in neurological patients, particularly those with spinal cord trauma or malformations of the spinal cord).

Voiding symptoms
- **Slow stream:** the perception of reduced urine flow, usually compared to previous performance or in comparison to others.
- **Splitting or spraying:** description of the urine stream.
- **Hesitancy:** difficulty in initiating micturition, resulting in a delay in the onset of voiding after the individual is ready to pass urine.
- **Intermittent stream (intermittency):** urine flow which stops and starts, on one or more occasions, during micturition.
- **Straining:** the muscular effort used to either initiate, maintain or improve the urinary stream.
- **Terminal dribble:** a prolonged final part of micturition, when the flow has slowed to a trickle/dribble (compare to post-micturition dribble).

Post-micturition symptoms
- **Feeling of incomplete emptying:** a feeling experienced by the individual after passing urine.
- **Post-micturition dribble:** the involuntary loss of urine immediately after an individual has finished passing urine, usually after leaving the toilet in men, or after rising from the toilet in women (compare to terminal dribble).

Other symptoms
- **Symptoms associated with sexual intercourse:** e.g. dyspareunia, vaginal dryness and incontinence (should be described as fully as possible – it is helpful to define urine leakage as: during penetration, during intercourse, or at orgasm).
- **Symptoms associated with pelvic organ prolapse:** e.g. 'something coming down', low backache, vaginal bulging sensation and dragging sensation (may need to digitally replace the prolapse in order to defaecate or micturate).
- **Genital and lower urinary tract pain:** pain, discomfort and pressure may be related to bladder filling or voiding or may be felt after micturition, or even be continuous. The terms 'strangury', 'bladder spasm', and 'dysuria' are difficult to define and of uncertain meaning and should not be used, unless a precise meaning is stated. Dysuria literally means 'abnormal urination'. However, it is often incorrectly used to describe the stinging/burning sensation characteristic of an urinary infection (UTI).

Painful bladder syndrome symptoms
- **Bladder pain syndrome/Painful bladder syndrome/interstitial cystitis (BPS/PBS/IC):** subrapubic pain related to bladder filling and associated with other lower urinary tract symptoms, usually increased frequency ((but not urgency) (diagnosed only in the absence of UTI or other obvious pathology)). This is a specific diagnosis usually confirmed by typical cystoscopic and histological features.

CHAPTER 2

Basic structure, function and control of the lower urinary tract

INTRODUCTION

The urinary tract consists of two distinct and mutually dependent components:

- upper tract – comprising the kidneys and ureters
- lower tract – comprising the urinary bladder and urethra.

These provide a highly sophisticated system of conduits and a reservoir that converts the continuous involuntary production of urine by the kidneys into the intermittent, consciously controlled voiding of urine (micturition at a convenient time and place).

A thorough understanding of the structure, function and control of the lower urinary tract is vital for the accurate interpretation of urodynamic investigations.

THE KIDNEYS AND URETERS

Both kidneys continuously produce greater than 0.5 ml of urine per kg of body weight per hour (i.e. >35 ml per hour in a 70 kg man) when functioning properly and adequately hydrated. This urine empties into the kidney's collecting systems which drain via the ureters.

The ureters function as low-pressure distensible conduits with intrinsic peristalsis, which transport urine from the kidneys to the bladder. The urine drains into the bladder at the vesico-ureteric junction (VUJ) at the termination of each ureter. Each junction if correctly functioning only allows the one way flow of urine and contains a mechanism to prevent retrograde transmission of urine back into the ureters from the bladder. This serves to protect the upper tract from the high pressures encountered within the bladder during voiding and to prevent infection entering the upper tracts.

THE URINARY BLADDER

The bladder is a hollow, muscular organ. It has two main functions:
- low pressure *storage* of urine
- *expulsion* of urine at an appropriate time and place.

Histologically the bladder is composed of three distinct layers:
1. **Serosa** – an outer adventitial connective tissue layer.
2. **Detrusor muscle** – a middle smooth muscle layer, comprising a functional syncytium of interlacing muscle bundles with fibres running in all directions.
3. **Urothelium** – an innermost lining composed of transitional cell epithelium providing an elastic barrier that is impervious to urine and which has a high metabolic rate and an important role in the control of bladder function (Figure 2.1).

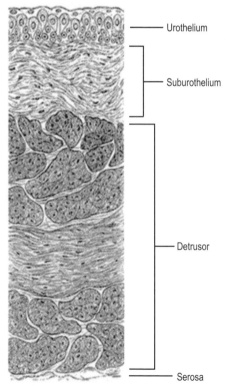

Figure 2.1 *Structure of the bladder wall.* The bladder wall is composed of four distinct layers and includes highly metabolically active urothelial and suburothelial layers.

4. **Suburothelial layer** – this lies immediately beneath the urothelim, is also highly active metabolically and acts in concert with the urothelium to subserve a key afferent role.

The base of the bladder extends circumferentially from the ureteric orifices. This region contains the trigone which is a small triangular muscular area between the two ureteric orifices and the bladder neck. The trigone contains a complex plexus of nerves. Above the ureteric orifices is the main body of the bladder.

THE URETHRA AND SPHINCTERIC MECHANISMS

The urethra has two main functions:
1. To provide an effective continence mechanism, for the majority of the time (storage phase).
2. To allow adequate emptying from the bladder with the minimum of resistance during micturition (voiding phase).

A further role for the urethra which seems likely but remains hypothetical is to provide afferent feedback which may have important implications in influencing bladder function. The innermost mucosal layer in both sexes is organized in longitudinal folds and during the storage phase when the urethra is 'closed' this appears in a stellate configuration on cross section. Such a configuration allows significant distensibility, which is necessary during urethral 'opening'.

The submucosal layer contains a vascular plexus which may be involved in improving the seal of a 'closed urethra' by transmitting the tension of the urethral muscle to the mucosal folds.

Apart from the obvious anatomical differences there are important differences in the configuration of the sphincter mechanisms between males and females (Figure 2.2).

Table 2.1 contrasts the longer urethra, a prostate and two powerful sphincter mechanisms in the male compared to the single weaker intrinsic sphincter mechanism with a weaker bladder neck and also a shorter urethra in the female.

Male sphincteric mechanisms

In the male there are two important sphincteric mechanisms:
1. A proximal 'bladder neck mechanism'.
2. A distal urethral mechanism at the apex of the prostate.

The proximal sphincter in the male bladder neck provides a powerful mechanism in both maintaining urinary continence and also preventing retrograde ejaculation of semen during sexual activity. In patients with a

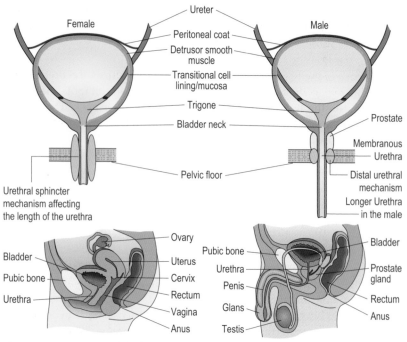

Figure 2.2 *Anatomy of the lower urinary tract in both sexes.*

Comparison of male and female sphincteric mechanisms

	Male	Female
Proximal bladder neck mechanism	Powerful	Weak
Distal urethral mechanism/urethral sphincter mechanism (in the female)	Powerful	Prone to the effect of exogenous influences such as pelvic floor weakness and damage or denervation consequent upon childbirth
Prostate	Further increases bladder outlet resistance	Not present
Urethra	Long	Short (~3.5 cm)

Table 2.1 *Comparison of male and female sphincteric mechanisms* – *showing why females are much more likely to develop an incompetent urethral mechanism and be prone to urinary incontinence from intrinsic sphincter deficiency (ISD).*

damaged distal urethral sphincter (e.g. a pelvic fracture-associated urethral disruption) continence can be maintained solely by the proximal bladder neck mechanism. Ultrastructurally it consists of a powerful inner layer of muscle bundles arranged in a circular orientation.

The distal sphincteric mechanism is also extremely important, as evidenced by its ability to maintain continence even when the proximal bladder neck mechanism has been rendered totally incompetent by surgical bladder neck incision or a prostatectomy. It is confined to the 3–5 mm thickness of the wall of the membranous urethra from the level of the verumontanum down to the distal aspect of the membranous urethra. It is composed mainly of extrinsic striated muscle which is capable of the sustained contraction necessary for continence and to a lesser degree by intrinsic smooth muscle.

Prostate gland

The prostate is made up of smooth muscle and glandular tissue, with the proportion of smooth muscle being increased in benign prostatic hyperplasia (BPH). The prostatic smooth muscle is controlled by the sympathetic nervous system, which acts by releasing noradrenaline onto α_{1a}-adrenoceptors located on the smooth muscle cells; the resulting contraction increases the bladder outlet resistance and further aids continence in the male.

Female sphincteric mechanisms

Females are much more likely to suffer from urinary incontinence due to sphincteric deficiency than males, due to the much less powerful sphincteric mechanisms. The bladder neck is a far weaker structure than the male bladder neck and is often incompetent, even in nulliparous young women. The bladder neck is poorly defined with the muscle fibres having a mainly longitudinal orientation.

Urinary continence is usually reliant upon the integrity of the urethral sphincteric mechanism, which like the male distal mechanism is composed of a longitudinal intrinsic urethral smooth muscle and a larger extrinsic striated muscle component. This sphincter extends throughout the proximal two-thirds of the urethra, being most developed in the middle one-third of the urethra. Damage to the sphincter or it's innervation (in particular the pudendal nerve) by obstetric trauma reduces the effectiveness of this mechanism and predisposes to stress urinary incontinence.

Pelvic floor muscles

In females the pelvic floor muscles also have an important role in maintaining continence. The pelvic floor is composed primarily of the levator ani muscle group, the endo-pelvic fascia and the supporting ligaments. The pelvic organs are maintained in the correct position by this pelvic floor. These tissues form a supporting 'hammock' beneath the urethra and during increases in intra-abdominal pressure (such as coughing, sneezing) the urethra is compressed against this hammock, thereby keeping the urethra closed and the patient continent (Figure 2.3).

Failure of this mechanism causes descent (prolapse) (Figure 2.4) and also hyper-mobility of the bladder neck and is an important cause of stress urinary incontinence (see Chapter 5).

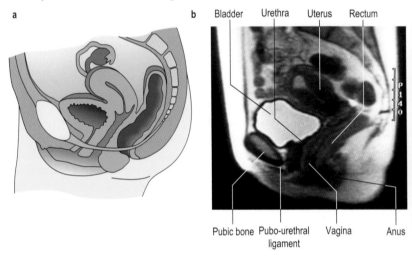

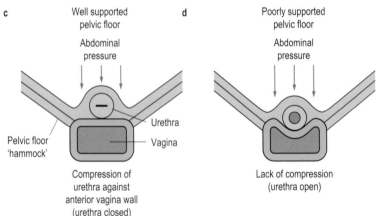

Figure 2.3 *Midline sagittal illustration of the female pelvis (a)* with corresponding MRI scan appearances *(b)*. Loss of pelvic floor (hammock) support *(c)*, causing a loss of transmission/compression of intra-abdominal pressure to the urethra.

Figure 2.4 *Prolapse of the bladder neck.* *Prolapsing bladder is clearly visible.*

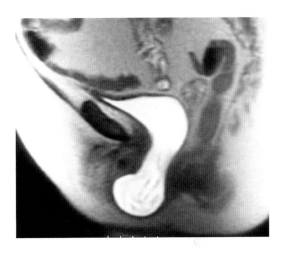

FUNCTION OF THE LOWER URINARY TRACT

The function of the lower urinary tract can be split into two distinct phases:

1. The storage (filling) phase.
2. The voiding phase.

For the majority of the time (greater than 99%) the lower urinary tract will be in the storage phase, whilst less than 1% of time is spent voiding.

Storage phase

During the storage phase the bladder is filled with urine from the ureters. The bladder needs to accommodate the increase in volume without an appreciable rise in bladder (intra-vesical) pressure. This receptive relaxation property is called the 'compliance' of the bladder. Factors that contribute to compliance are:

- The passive elastic properties of the tissues of the bladder wall.
- The intrinsic ability of smooth muscle to maintain a constant tension over a wide range of stretch.
- The neural reflexes which control detrusor tension during bladder filling.

During the storage phase the urethra and sphincteric mechanisms should be closed, thereby maintaining a high outlet resistance and continence.

13

Voiding phase

During the voiding phase the reverse activity to that seen during the storage phase must occur. The bladder must cease relaxing and instead contract to expel the urine and the urethra and sphincteric mechanisms must 'open' to decrease the outlet resistance and allow passage of urine. Voiding should be efficient and there should be minimal or no urine remaining in the bladder at the end of the voiding phase.

During voiding:
1. Urethral relaxation precedes detrusor contraction.
2. Simultaneous relaxation of the pelvic floor muscles occurs.
3. 'Funnelling' of the bladder neck occurs to facilitate flow of urine into the proximal urethra.
4. Detrusor contraction occurs to forcefully expel urine.

Return to storage phase

At the end of voiding the proximal urethra is closed in a retrograde fashion, thus milking back the urine into the bladder. This 'milkback' is seen during contrast studies of the lower urinary tract when the patient is asked to stop voiding. Following this the bladder returns to a state of relaxation.

URODYNAMICS IN PRACTICE

Storage phase
- Bladder fills passively – detrusor muscle is relaxed.
- Urethral sphincter mechanisms are 'closed' – urethral and pelvic floor muscles are contracted.

Voiding phase
- Bladder actively expels urine under conscious voluntary control – detrusor muscle is contracting.
- Urethral sphincter mechanisms are 'open' – urethral and pelvic floor muscles are relaxed.

NEURONAL CONTROL OF THE LOWER URINARY TRACT

Control of the lower urinary tract is executed via a complex series of peripheral and central neuronal pathways. These pathways:
- co-ordinate the activities of the bladder and the urethral/sphincter mechanisms
- control receptive relaxation of the bladder (compliance)

- sense bladder fullness
- maintain continence with increasing fullness of the bladder
- initiate voluntary voiding.

Motor (efferent) control

- The storage phase is under predominant sympathetic control.
- The voiding phase is under predominant parasympathetic control.

The peripheral innervation of the lower urinary tract is principally from three groups of nerves (Table 2.2 and Figure 2.5):
1. hypogastric
2. pelvic
3. pudendal.

Sensory (afferent) control

Afferent signalling from the lower urinary tract also occurs along the hypogastric, pelvic and pudendal nerves. These nerves transmit information regarding the fullness of the bladder as well as the presence of any noxious (chemical or cold) stimuli.

The principal innervations of the lower urinary tract

	Type	Origin	Detrusor muscle	Sphincteric muscle	Principal neurotransmitter
Hypogastric	Sympathetic	T10–L2	Relaxes	Contracts sphincteric smooth muscle	Noradrenaline
Pelvic	Parasympathetic	S2–S4 (spinal micturition centre)	Contracts	Relaxes	Acetylcholine
Pudendal	Somatic	S2–S4 (Onuf's nucleus)	N/A	Contracts sphincteric striated muscle and pelvic floor	Acetylcholine

Table 2.2 *The principal innervation of the lower urinary tract.*

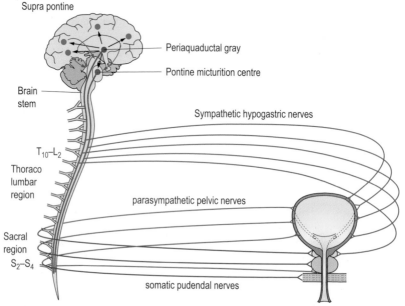

Figure 2.5 Neural control of the lower urinary tract. *Showing the somatic, sympathetic and parasympathetic peripheral nerves; the pontine micturition centre, the periaqueductal gray and the suprapontine areas involved in control of storage and voiding of urine. There are extensive interactions at all levels (not shown).*

Afferent signalling is involved in:

- involuntary reflexes
- conscious sensation of bladder fullness.

In certain neurogenic or inflammatory conditions there is up-regulation of some of these afferent nerves, causing bladder pain and it is thought that type C afferent nerve fibres are implicated in the involuntary stimulation of detrusor contractions (detrusor overactivity).

Involuntary storage reflexes

A number of involuntary reflexes exist, which are mainly located in the lumbo-sacral spinal cord. With increasing bladder fullness these reflexes will increase sympathetic activity and inhibit parasympathetic activity and also activate the pudendal (somatic) neurones. These reflexes therefore enhance storage by relaxing the bladder and maintain continence by increasing both intrinsic and extrinsic sphincter tone (guarding reflex).

Voiding reflexes are not confined to the spinal cord and there are a number of supra-spinal reflexes involved in co-ordinating lower urinary tract activity that have been discovered in experimentally produced high spinal cord transections.

Desire to void

After infancy, voluntary control of voiding is achieved, thus allowing voiding to be initiated only in appropriate circumstances. To achieve this, information regarding bladder fullness must be sent to the brain, and when appropriate to void the brain must override the peripheral storage reflexes and 'switch' the lower urinary tract into the voiding phase.

Once a threshold level of fullness has been achieved (which will depend upon circumstances and vary between individuals) there will be increasing afferent activity emanating from sensory neurones in the suburothelial plexus associated with the bladder wall. Parasympathetic afferents in the pelvic nerve will communicate this activity via the spinal cord to the peri-aqueductal gray (PAG) area in the midbrain. At the PAG the bladder filling information is processed and from here the signals are sent to the pontine micturition centre (PMC) in the brainstem and the suprapontine areas of the brain.

The suprapontine areas of the brain comprises the frontal cortex, the hypothalamus, the para-central lobule, the limbic system and the cingulate gyrus. These are important in the conscious and unconscious control of the PMC. They have a role in delaying micturition, inhibiting premature detrusor contractions and in initiating voiding at an appropriate time.

Voluntary control of voiding

The PMC is an essential control centre in co-ordinating the micturition process and is itself under the control of the suprapontine area.

If the bladder is sensed to be full but it is inappropriate to void then the PMC will send descending signals to inhibit parasympathetic activity, increase sympathetic activity and increase the pudendal somatic activity to contract the urethral sphincter mechanism and pelvic floor muscles. These mechanisms voluntarily 'tighten up' the bladder outlet and so maintain continence until an appropriate time and place is found to void.

If the bladder is sensed to be full and it is appropriate to void then the PMC will 'switch' the lower urinary tract into the voiding phase by sending descending signals to increase parasympathetic activity and inhibit sympathetic and somatic activity.

Once voiding is initiated, secondary reflexes in the urethra, activated by urine flow also further facilitate bladder emptying.

Neuronal interactions

The account of the neuronal control of the lower urinary tract given above is a simplification; there are extensive interactions between the neuronal populations at all levels in both the peripheral, spinal and higher central areas. These complex neuronal interactions have led to much controversy regarding the motor control of the lower urinary tract and also more recently regarding the sensory feedback. In particular the role of the sub-urothelial layer in afferent feedback involving a variety of neurotransmitters is currently the focus of much research. In recent years it has been recognised that stretch of the urothelial mucosa can lead to the non-neuronal release of a number of neurotransmitters such as acetylcholine, nitric oxide and ATP. In addition, an important group of cells, so called 'interstitial cells' have also been identified and these undoubtedly have an important role in the coordination of lower urinary tract function. This remains an evolving area with continuing research into the mechanisms underpinning lower urinary tract function.

CONCLUSIONS

A broad understanding of lower urinary tract function and its control is vital to accurately interpret urodynamic investigations and in understanding the pathophysiology and treatment of urinary tract disorders such as incontinence, bladder outlet obstruction and neurogenic dysfunction.

CHAPTER 3

Urodynamic procedures

INTRODUCTION

Symptomatic evaluation of urinary tract dysfunction is difficult since the bladder often proves to be an 'unreliable witness', not only because of subjective bias from both the patient and the clinician; but also because there is considerable overlap between the symptoms from different disorders. Urodynamic techniques are objective investigations developed to clarify these symptoms. The term urodynamics encompasses a variety of complementary techniques of varying complexity (Table 3.1).

In this chapter the indications and methodology for these various techniques will be discussed along with introducing common clinical findings. The majority of invasive urodynamic investigations are pressure/flow studies and these will be discussed in detail in the next chapter (Chapter 4). More detailed discussion of common lower urinary tract disorders and associated urodynamic findings will occur in later chapters.

INDICATIONS FOR URODYNAMIC ASSESSMENTS

Only a good understanding of the various techniques including methodology, limitations and specific indications will allow the clinician to choose an appropriate test. In many cases a number of investigations may be necessary to answer all the clinical questions or further investigations may be required if the first investigation was unhelpful or presents a new avenue for investigation.

Before embarking on any urodynamic investigation the following should be considered:
- Is there a clear indication for the chosen test?
  - Will it aid in diagnosis?
  - Will it aid in making management decisions?
- Is this the most appropriate test?
  - Would a simpler test answer the clinical questions?
  - Is a more complex test more likely to answer *all* the clinical questions?

Urodynamic techniques	
Complexity of technique	**Technique**
Simple – voiding diary	Micturition/time chart Frequency/volume chart Bladder diary
Simple – investigation	Pad testing Uroflowmetry ± ultrasound residual Ultrasound cystodynamogram Intravenous urodynamogram
Pressure/flow studies (Chapter 4)	Cystometry Leak point measurements Video urodynamics Ambulatory urodynamics
Complex – investigation	Urethral pressure measurement Neuro-physiological investigation Upper tract urodynamics (Whitaker test)

Table 3.1 *Urodynamic techniques.*

- Are there appropriate local facilities and expertise to perform the chosen test?
- Is the most appropriate person, with an understanding of the patient's individual condition performing the test?

STANDARDIZATION AND QUALITY CONTROL

All urodynamics should be performed in a standardized manner; this not only maintains the quality of the data, but also allows for comparison of the results if a patient has a repeat investigation. In addition a standardized technique and recording of the data using recognized terminology allows the accurate exchange and comparison of information for both clinical and experimental purposes. The official terminology suggested by the International Continence Society (ICS) is used throughout this book. However investigations must still be tailored for individual patients so that the clinical questions are answered thoroughly without undue time spent on obtaining clinically irrelevant data.

Maintaining the quality of any study also requires that all equipment is appropriately set up and regularly calibrated with sufficient working knowledge to 'troubleshoot' any problems encountered during an investigation.

In all cases precise measurement and complete documentation must be coupled with accurate analysis and critical reporting of the results. However, it must be borne in mind that whilst these are objective tests that can be standardized to a high degree, there remains a significant subjective element in the interpretation of the results. Urodynamics is not an exact science!

AIMS OF URODYNAMIC INVESTIGATIONS

The principal aim of any urodynamic assessment is to reproduce the symptoms whilst obtaining physiological measurements, so as to determine the pathophysiology underlying the symptoms.

Both the precise nature of the condition and the severity can be established, thus allowing the clinician to understand the clinical implications and plan further appropriate management.

URODYNAMICS IN PRACTICE

Aims of urodynamic investigations:
- Reproduce the troublesome symptoms.
- Answer specific clinical questions.
- Establish a precise diagnosis.
- Determine the severity of the condition.
- Plan further investigations or therapies.

In most cases the indications for urodynamic investigation are clear and its appropriate application is essential to the modern practice of urology, gynaecology, and any specialties dealing with the management of lower urinary tract dysfunction.

CLINICAL NOTES

Always exclude urinary tract infections prior to an urodynamic investigation
- Urinary tract infections (UTIs) are a common cause of LUTS.
- A UTI may aggravate pre-existing LUTS.
- The presence of a UTI may invalidate the results of a urodynamic investigation, as a UTI may falsely result in:
  - increased bladder sensation (± pain or discomfort)
  - detrusor overactivity
  - poor bladder compliance.
- Prophylactic antibiotics may play a role in patients with recurrent UTIs, allowing the study to be performed with sterile urine.

VOIDING DIARIES

Voiding diaries are the simplest of all urodynamic assessments, yet their value is often overlooked. They provide an important natural urodynamic record of bladder function.

Indications and aims

Voiding diaries are simple, non-invasive tools that are frequently part of the initial evaluation of patients complaining of LUTS, particularly those who have storage symptoms such as increased urinary frequency and incontinence.

They give an indication of the voiding pattern, the severity of symptoms and they add objectivity to the history. They may also give an indication of the impact on the patient's life and may highlight 'coping strategies' that the patient has adopted to help manage their symptoms. Voiding diaries are also useful in identifying pathophysiology of renal origin such as abnormal production of urine related to the circadian rhythm.

A number of different diaries have been defined by the ICS:

- **Micturition time chart** – records only the times that voids occur with no volumetric data.
- **Frequency/volume chart (FVC)** – records the time and volume of each micturition.
- **Bladder diary** – records the time and volume of each micturition and may also include other data such as incontinence episodes, pad usage, fluid intake and urgency (Table 3.2).

Method and standardization

The patient is asked to record as accurately as possible the time of events such as voids and incontinent episodes on the chart and to measure the volume voided using a graduated container (jug). They are also asked to record the time they are awake and asleep. Patients must be instructed to continue their normal activities during the course of the assessment, so as to obtain an accurate representation of their normal lower urinary tract function. The ICS has recommended that voiding diaries are performed for at least 24 hours, although in practice a period of 3–7 days is usually chosen. Most patients find them acceptable for use over short periods.

Bladder diary

Week Commencing: / /

	Monday		Tuesday		Wednesday		Thursday		Friday		Saturday		Sunday	
	In	Out	In	Out	In	Out	In	Out	In	Out	In	Out	In	Out
6am	300				350						200		190	
7am			200				250		350		100			170
8am		50				150				250		190		
9am	250	150	100				150							
10am					150			200					100	
11am	175	100			175				200		180			
12.00				250		100						150		130
1pm							200			200				
2pm	190	W		130	150			175					270	
3pm						W			100	W	270			
4pm								W						
5pm	300	200				150	200			150		W		W
6pm				190	200									
7pm		75		W				150				100	180	
8pm						100			200	175				
9pm	150	100											120	
10pm				150					175		190			175
11pm							100		100					
12.00				50	W		100				100			
1am													100	
2am		W							W		W			120
3am					120									
4am														
5am			150											
Waking	6am		7.45am		7.30am		7.00am		6.30am		7.45am		7.40am	
Retiring	12.30am		11.30pm		12.51am		Midnight		Midnight		12.30am		11.30pm	
Pad usage	3		1		2		4		3		5		2	

Table 3.2 Bladder diary. *Recording volume and time of each void, fluid intake, pad usage and incontinence episodes (W). Patients also record waking/retiring time to allow calculation of nocturia.*

Frequent findings

- Normal frequency and voided volumes.
- Increased frequency and normal volumes – therefore an increased 24-hour production of urine, suggesting a high fluid intake. This may be related to diabetes mellitus or diabetes insipidus but is more usually habitual, especially with the increasing popularity of high fluid diets.
- Reduced volumes with minimal variation in the volume voided – suggesting a bladder wall pathology such as bladder pain syndrome/painful bladder syndrome/interstitial cystitis or carcinoma in situ (Note – An anatomical capacity measured under general anaesthesia will confirm the presence of a reduced bladder capacity due to anatomical reasons such as fibrosis or a contracted bladder. A reduced anatomical capacity often implies a low likelihood of response to conservative therapeutic modalities).
- Reduced volumes with variation in the volume voided – suggestive of underlying detrusor overactivity as the bladder contracts at variable degrees of distension before maximum capacity, erroneously informing the patient that it is full; resulting in urinary frequency and low and variable voided volumes.
- Increased nocturnal production – (nocturnal polyuria), suggestive of cardiac failure, dependent fluid shifts in the supine position, hormonal fluid balance abnormality or idiopathic in origin. This is not a urological condition.

Voiding diaries must not be over-interpreted, but should be used in combination with other forms of urodynamic and urological assessment (Table 3.3).

Bladder retraining

In addition to having diagnostic benefit, voiding diaries have therapeutic value and can provide important information that is helpful in treating bladder dysfunction. It is particularly useful for providing biofeedback during bladder retraining drills commonly used in patients with small volume frequency and urgency incontinence. They also often provide important feedback to the practitioner and patient so that they can objectively evaluate the effectiveness of any therapy.

Urodynamic parameters measured by voiding diaries

Daytime frequency	Number of voids recorded in waking hours
Nocturia	Number of voids recorded during sleep hours with each void preceded and followed by sleep
24-hour frequency	Total number of awake and sleep voids during a specified 24-hour period
24-hour production	Total volume of urine voided during a specified 24-hour period
Polyuria	Voiding of more than 2.8 litres in 24 hours
Nocturnal urine volume	Total volume of urine voided during sleep hours, excluding the last void before sleeping but including the first void on waking
Nocturnal polyuria	When an increased proportion of the 24-hour production occurs at night, usually >33% (but age-dependent)
Maximum voided volume (replaces the term 'functional volume')	The largest volume voided during a single micturition. Particularly important when deciding how much to fill the bladder during pressure/flow urodynamics, to prevent overfilling
Pad usage	Number of pads used during a specified period
Frequency of incontinence episodes	Number of incontinence episodes during a specified period
Frequency of urgency episodes	Number of urgency episodes during a specified period
Fluid intake	Volume of fluid ingested during a specified period

Table 3.3 *Urodynamic parameters measured by voiding diaries.*

CLINICAL NOTES

Example of bladder retraining programme
In order to bring your bladder problem under control you must re-educate your bladder and learn to resist early false sensations of bladder fullness. Retraining (or 'stretching') your bladder will help to control leakage and you can do this by trying to hold on for as long as possible before passing water.

- It is important that you **do not** restrict your fluid intake.
- When you get the feeling that you need to pass urine, **suppress the urge until the sensation lessens or subsides.**
- At first this will be difficult but as you persevere it will become easier.

- Sitting on a hard seat may help you to hold on to your urine for longer. Helpful distractors include taking deep breaths, counting backwards from 100, etc.
- Contracting the pelvic floor muscles (Kegel manoeuvre) can also help to abort the desire to void.
- If you wake up at night, try to hold on if you can; if possible, turn over and go back to sleep.
- If you have been prescribed tablets to help you pass your urine less frequently take them regularly as directed.
- You should aim to reduce the frequency with which you pass urine to five or six times in 24 hours.

Remember:
You are trying to re-educate your bladder so that it will hold more urine. Although you may find this difficult at first, with practice it will get easier.

Example of bladder drill
Patients are instructed to:
- hold on to their urine for a fixed time, such as an hour
- Use the bladder retraining programme to suppress early urges
- and gradually increase the time interval (for instance, an additional 15 minutes weekly) between voids until an acceptable voiding pattern is achieved.

Pad testing

Pad testing is a simple, non-invasive and objective method for detecting and quantifying urinary incontinence. It is easy to perform and interpret and provides a great deal of useful information.

Indications and aims

The principal aim is to determine the amount of urine leaked during a specified period, e.g. one hour, thus quantifying the severity of incontinence to both clinician and patient, as frequently the degree of incontinence is unclear from the history. In addition, the test is particularly useful to confirm the presence of incontinence when other tests, e.g. pressure/flow urodynamics, have failed to demonstrate any urinary leakage.

Method and standardization

To obtain a representative result, especially for those who have variable or intermittent urinary incontinence, the test period should be as long as possible in circumstances that approximate to those of everyday life; yet it must be practical. The pad test should be conducted in a standardized fashion and the ICS have provided guidelines on performing a '1-hour pad test'.

URODYNAMICS IN PRACTICE: 1-HOUR PAD TEST

The International Continence Society has suggested the following guidelines:

- The test should occupy a 1-hour period during which a series of standard activities are carried out.
- The test can be extended by further 1-hour periods if the result of the first 1-hour test is not considered to be representative by either the patient or the investigator; alternatively the test can be repeated after filling the bladder to a defined volume.
- The total amount of urine leaked during the test period is determined by weighing a collecting device such as a nappy, absorbent pad, or condom appliance (ensure that the collecting device has adequate capacity).
- A nappy or pad should be worn inside waterproof underpants or should have a waterproof backing.
- Immediately before the test begins the collecting device is weighed to the nearest gram.

Typical test schedule

- Test is started without the patient voiding.
- Pre-weighed collecting device (pad) is put on and first 1-hour test period begins.
- Patient drinks 500 ml sodium-free liquid within a short period (maximum 15 min), then sits or rests.
- Patient walks for 30 min, including stair climbing equivalent to one flight up and down.
- For remaining period the patient performs the following activities: standing up from sitting, 10 times; coughing vigorously, 10 times; running on the spot for 1 min; bending to pick up small object from floor, 5 times; washes hands in running water for 1 min.
- At the end of the 1-hour test the collecting device is removed and weighed. The change of weight of the collecting device is recorded. A change of less than 1 g is within experimental error and the patient should be regarded as essentially dry.
- If the test is regarded as representative the subject voids and the volume is recorded, otherwise the test is repeated preferably without voiding.
- If the collecting device becomes saturated or filled during the test it should be removed and weighed, and replaced by a fresh device.
- The activity programme may be modified according to the patient's physical ability.

Practical points

- The total weight of urine lost during the test period is taken to be equal to the gain in weight of the collecting device(s). An increase in weight of the pad of less than 1 g in 1 hour is not considered to be a sign of incontinence, as such as small weight change may be due to weighing errors, sweating, or vaginal discharge.
- The test should not be performed during a menstrual period.
- A negative result should be interpreted with caution; the test may need to be repeated or supplemented with a more prolonged test.
- Any variations from the usual test schedule should be recorded, so that the same schedule can be used on subsequent occasions.
- In principle, patients should not void during the test period. If they experience urgency, they should be persuaded to postpone voiding and to perform as many of the activities listed for the last 15–30 min of the test as possible to detect leakage.
- Before voiding the collection device is removed for weighing. Patients may influence the test result by voiding prior to removing and weighing the pad.
- If voiding cannot be postponed the test is terminated. The voided volume and duration of the test should be recorded. The results for patients who are unable to complete the test may require separate analysis or the test may be repeated after rehydration.

Urodynamic parameters measured by pad testing

Pad testing determines the volume of leakage during a specified period. One gram is equal to one millilitre, therefore an increase in weight of the collection device (pad) by for example 10 g is equal to urinary incontinence of 10 ml.

Normal values

The hourly pad weight increase in continent women varies from 0.0 to 2.1 g/hour, averaging 0.26 g/hour. With the 1-hour International Continence Society pad test, the upper limit (99% confidence limit) has been found to be 1.4 g/hour.

URODYNAMICS IN PRACTICE: VARIATIONS TO THE PAD TEST

- Colouration of the urine with oral pyridium before pad testing can help differentiate between vaginal discharge and urinary incontinence.
- Additional changes and weighing of the collecting device can give information about the timing of urine loss.
- The collecting device may be an electronic recording pad so that the timing is recorded directly.
- Home pad tests lasting 24–48 hours are superior to 1-hour tests in detecting urinary incontinence. However they are less practical and more cumbersome. The pads must be stored in an airtight container before and after use to prevent evaporation, until they have been weighed. The normal upper limit for a 24-hour test is 8 g.
- Experts who routinely perform pad testing do so for a number of reasons:
  - severe patients with high volume incontinence may experience lower cure rates with anti-incontinence procedures
  - pad testing provides an excellent objective outcome measure.

UROFLOWMETRY

This is the simplest and often most useful investigation in the assessment of patients with predominantly voiding symptoms.

Indications and aims

This is a non-invasive and inexpensive test that gives a great deal of information regarding voiding function by measuring the rate of flow of voided urine.

- It can often be used to support the diagnosis of bladder outlet obstruction (BOO) or a poorly functioning detrusor, suspected from the history.
- It is an excellent screening tool for BOO, particularly when combined with measurement of residual urine volume and is frequently the first line screening investigation for most patients with suspected voiding dysfunction.
- It is useful for identifying those patients who require more extensive urodynamic evaluation.

Uroflowmetry is an adequate investigation for uncomplicated BOO in over 60% of patients. More detailed investigations are only indicated in limited situations, such as when the findings are at variance with the symptoms, if there are significant storage symptoms or if initial treatment has been unsuccessful.

Method and standardization

Uroflowmetry is performed using a flowmeter, a device that measures the quantity of fluid (volume or mass) voided per unit time (Figure 3.1). The measurement is expressed in millilitres per second (ml/s). Patients are instructed to void normally, either sitting or standing, with a comfortably full bladder and should be provided with as much privacy as possible and comfortable surroundings, so as to remove the inhibitory effects of the test environment. Uroflowmetry can be carried out either by itself or in combination with other techniques such as the measurement of post-void residual (PVR) urine. The patient should be asked if the void was representative of their usual voiding. (It is important that the flowmeter is regularly calibrated as per the manufacturer's instructions to maintain the accuracy of the readings.)

URODYNAMICS IN PRACTICE: TYPES OF FLOWMETER

- **Rotating disk flowmeter:** the voided fluid is directed onto a rotating disk and the amount landing on the disk produces a proportionate increase in its inertia; the power required to keep the disk rotating at a constant rate is measured, so allowing calculation of the flow rate of fluid landing on the disk.
- **Electronic dipstick flowmeter:** a dipstick is mounted in a collecting chamber and as urine accumulates the electrical capacitance of the dipstick changes, allowing calculation of the rate of fluid accumulation and hence the flow rate.
- **Gravimetric flowmeter:** the weight of collected fluid or the hydrostatic pressure at the base of a collecting cylinder is measured. The change in weight or pressure allows calculation of the flow rate.

Normal values

Males under 40 years of age generally have maximum flow rates over 25 ml/s. Flow rates decrease with age and men over 60 years of age with no bladder outlet obstruction usually have maximum flow rates over 15 ml/s.

Females have higher flow rates than males, usually of the order of 5–10 ml/s more for a given bladder volume. Exaggerated maximum flow rates are typical in women who have stress incontinence, where the outlet resistance is minimal and also in patients who have marked detrusor overactivity – the so-called 'fast bladder'.

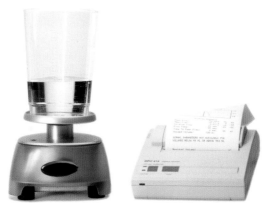

Figure 3.1 Flowmeter. *Photograph of a typical flowmeter which is usually placed below a large funnel for the patient to void into. The funnel is normally placed under a commode for females; men can void directly into the funnel whilst standing. Photograph also shows results printer.*

Interpretation

Uroflowmetry is invaluable in the assessment of voiding function for a wide range of urological conditions. Reliance should be placed on the observed flow pattern as well as any absolute values obtained (Figures 3.2 and 3.3). The results must always be interpreted within the context of the clinical situation, recognizing the limitations of the study.

The measured flow rate is dependent upon a number of factors including:

- strength of detrusor contraction (detrusor contractility)
- presence of bladder outlet obstruction (BOO)
- adequacy of relaxation of the sphincter mechanisms
- patency of the urethra
- compensatory mechanisms such as abdominal straining.

The flow rate and pattern give important clues as to the underlying dysfunction, however the major limitation of uroflowmetry is that the flow rate is a composite of both the function of the detrusor and the function of the bladder outlet/urethra. It is therefore impossible to determine from a flow rate alone if voiding dysfunction is due to a detrusor pathology or bladder outlet/urethral pathology or from a combination of problems; only pressure/flow urodynamics can differentiate between such conditions. For example, prolonged flow time with an abnormally low Q_{max} may be due to bladder outlet/urethral obstruction or a poorly contractile detrusor muscle (detrusor underactivity). However, a number of charac-

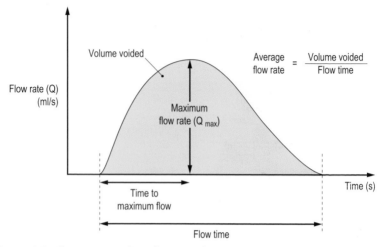

Figure 3.2 *Flow rate recording.* Illustrating the International Continence Society nomenclature. (Reproduced with permission from Neurourology and Urodynamics 1988; 7:403–426.)

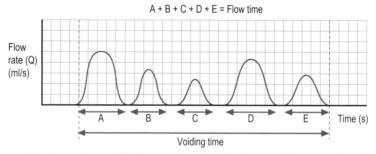

Figure 3.3 *Intermittent void.* Showing the relationship between flow time and voiding time in an intermittent voiding pattern.

teristic uroflowmetry patterns have been described, and whilst these may not be specific, in the majority of patients they give an acceptable indication of the most likely pathology and allow empirical therapy to be instigated (Table 3.4).

Characteristic flow patterns

Normal – An easily distensible bladder outlet with a normal detrusor contraction results in a smooth bell-shaped curve with a rapid rise to a high

Urodynamic parameters measured by uroflowmetry

Parameter	Definition	Notes
Voided volume	Total volume expelled via the urethra	
Maximum flow rate (Q_{max})	Maximum measured flow rate	The flow curve should be assessed visually and the Q_{max} must not be taken at the peak of an artefact but at the peak of the line of best fit for the curve
Average flow rate	Voided volume divided by flow time	Calculation of average flow rate is only meaningful if flow is continuous and without terminal dribbling
Flow time	Time over which measurable flow actually occurs (i.e. excluding interruptions)	The flow pattern must be described when flow time and average flow rate are measured
Voiding time	Total duration of micturition (i.e. including interruptions)	When voiding is completed without interruption, voiding time is equal to flow time
Time to maximum flow	Elapsed time from onset of flow to maximum flow rate	

Table 3.4 *Urodynamic parameters measured by uroflowmetry.*

amplitude peak (Q_{max}). The time to Q_{max} should not exceed one-third of the flow time. Any other patterns (flat, multiple peaks, asymmetric, prolonged) indicate abnormal voiding (Figure 3.4a).

'Fast bladder' – This is an exaggeration of the normal curve and may be due to a raised end fill bladder pressure associated with detrusor overactivity or may be due to a significant decrease in outflow resistance as can occur with stress urinary incontinence (Figure 3.4b).

Prolonged flow – This is a flow with a prolonged time to reach a low maximum amplitude and an extended flow time; often it is an asymmetric curve with a prolonged declining terminal end. This is frequently seen with bladder outlet obstruction (BOO), although a similar pattern may be seen with a poorly contractile detrusor muscle (Figure 3.4c).

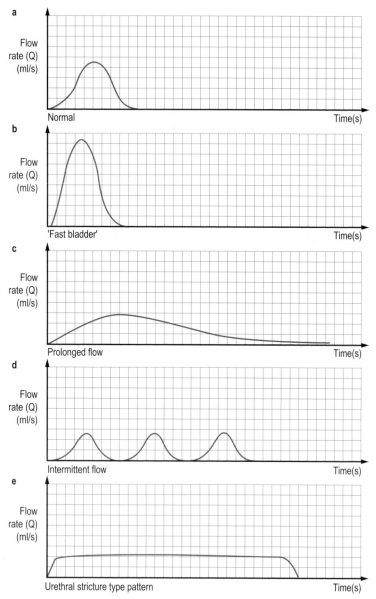

Figure 3.4 *Characteristic flow patterns.* (**a**) Normal – there is rapid change before and after the peak flow. (**b**) 'Fast bladder' – an exaggeration of normal associated with high pre-micturition pressure and seen in cases of detrusor overactivity. (**c**) Prolonged flow – associated with outflow obstruction. (**d**) Intermittent flow – resulting from abdominal straining to compensate for poor detrusor contractility; a similar picture may be seen with urethral overactivity (detrusor sphincter dyssynergia or dysfunctional voiding). (**e**) Classical pattern of a urethral stricture with a long plateau.

Intermittent flow – This irregular spiking pattern is frequently due to abdominal straining to overcome the poor flow associated with BOO or a poorly contractile detrusor, although more complex outlet conditions such as sporadic sphincter activity may also cause an intermittent pattern (Figure 3.4d).

Flat plateau – A low maximum flow rate which plateaus for a prolonged time in a 'box-like' fashion is characteristic of a constrictive obstruction from a urethral stricture. A urethral stricture in the presence of a normally functioning bladder usually does not cause voiding symptoms until the urethral calibre is reduced below 11 F (Figure 3.4e).

To provide more detailed information a simple flow rate can be combined with a measurement of the post-voiding residual (PVR) volume. If there is doubt about the diagnosis after uroflowmetry, more complex urodynamic (usually pressure/flow) studies may be required. For instance, it may be ill-advised to perform a prostatectomy in men with lower urinary tract symptoms (LUTS) who have a normal flow pattern, a 'fast bladder', or very intermittent flow and a high PVR, without first performing pressure/flow urodynamics.

Practical points

There are a number of important factors to consider when interpreting flow rates including:

- Volume voided – low voided volumes of <150 ml can lead to erroneous results and should be repeated; whereas high voided volumes of >400–600 ml may lower flow rates by overstretching the bladder, resulting in detrusor overdistension and decompensation (Note – Many patients complain of slower flow rates at night when the bladder is relatively overstretched).
- The nature of the fluid – flowmeters need to be calibrated for the type of fluid being voided, due to differences in specific gravity.
- Age and sex – as these may alter the flow rates.
- Pattern – in particular whether the flow is continuous or intermittent.
- Position of the patient when voiding – should be noted, e.g. sitting, standing, supine.
- Free flow – a 'free flow' occurs after natural filling of the bladder, whereas a 'non free flow' void occurs when the bladder is filled using a catheter. The 'free flow' void is more physiological.

CLINICAL NOTES

Note: normal flow rate does not rule out bladder outlet obstruction (BOO)

Frequently uroflowmetry is performed to detect the presence and severity of BOO. However, particularly in the early stages of obstruction there may be a compensatory increase in the voiding pressure generated by the detrusor muscle, thus overcoming the obstruction. Uroflowmetry may therefore be normal in the presence of BOO. Pressure/flow urodynamics can detect the BOO in such a situation. This high pressure, normal flow voiding (>15 ml/s) occurs in approximately 7–15% of patients with bladder outflow obstruction.

A Q_{max} of <12 mL/s is generally considered abnormal in men >60 years; data suggest that approximately 90% of men with LUTS and a Q_{max} <10 mL/s are obstructed on pressure/flow studies.

Artefacts

The maximum flow rate recorded by the uroflowmetry machine is frequently misleading. Common artefacts are shown in Figure 3.5 and include:

- Straining, causing an artificial rise in the maximum flow rate.
- Irregularities in the measured flow rate due to collecting funnel artefacts and variations in direction of the urinary stream. Such as occurs when a man voiding into a funnel changes the point he is 'aiming' at within the funnel.

Due to the kinetics of smooth muscle contraction the detrusor is unable to generate short lived changes in amplitude (spikes). Therefore these artefacts need to be removed by the clinician by examining the pattern and 'smoothing' the curve with a line of best fit to determine the actual Q_{max}. *It is incorrect to blindly assume that the electronically reported Q_{max} is accurate.*

It must also be remembered that any alteration in the urinary stream after the urine leaves the meatus may alter the flow and introduce artefacts. The funnel/collecting device will invariably cause such modifications. There is also a lag in the flowmeter registering the flow from when the urine left the meatus; this is unimportant in free flow uroflowmetry but is a consideration when uroflowmetry is combined with pressure/flow urodynamics (see Chapter 4).

The pattern of the flow is also altered by the speed of the recording and the ICS have recommended that:

- 1 millimetre should equal 1 second on the x-axis
- 1 millimetre should equal 10 millilitres on the y-axis.

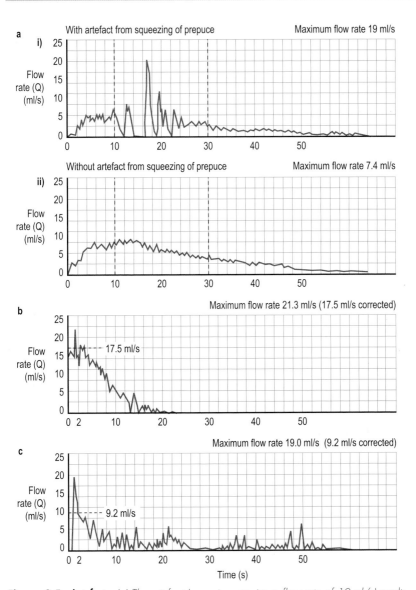

Figure 3.5 Artefacts. (**a**) The artefact (a spurious maximum flow rate of 19 ml/s) results from squeezing the prepuce of the penis during voiding. (**b**) It is eliminated revealing a true maximum flow rate of 7.4 ml/s when the patient stops squeezing the penis. (**c** and **d**) Both these flow curves show artefactual spikes, but an experienced urologist has corrected the traces (dotted line) so that the true maximum flow rates are 17.5 and 9.2 ml/s, as shown. Frequently an artefactual spike occurs at the start of the recorded flow due to the initial flow of urine registering on the flowmeter; or during the flow pattern due to abdominal straining.

POST-VOID RESIDUAL (PVR) DETERMINATION

Frequently uroflowmetry is combined with simple post-void residual (PVR) estimation using a handheld ultrasonic 'bladder scanner' to estimate the completeness of bladder emptying. When more information on bladder anatomy and function is needed an ultrasound cystodynamogram can be performed (see next section).

An elevated post-void residual (PVR) may represent obstruction; or more commonly is a surrogate marker for detrusor failure which may be due to a number of causes, including chronic BOO, neurogenic bladder or myogenic failure. An elevated PVR is an indication for pressure/flow urodynamics.

There are a number of clinical implications of an elevated PVR:

- may be an indication for prostatectomy in obstructed male patients
- requires long-term surveillance in those followed conservatively
- may be associated with hydronephrosis
- predisposes patient to recurrent urinary tract infections and bladder calculi
- potential risk factor for retention in patients managed with antimuscarinic agents.

ULTRASOUND CYSTODYNAMOGRAM

The ultrasound cystodynamogram (USCD) combines ultrasound examination of the bladder with uroflowmetry to provide more detailed information on bladder structure and function than uroflowmetry alone.

Indications and aims

Additional information obtained during an USCD includes the structure of the bladder (shape, presence of diverticulia), distal ureteric anatomy (presence of hydroureteronephrosis), completeness of bladder emptying and the prostate size (Figure 3.6).

An USCD is of particular value for assessing patients who may have a raised PVR (e.g. patients with suspected outflow obstruction, a poorly functioning detrusor or if there is suspected compromised voiding after a repair procedure for stress incontinence).

The addition of ultrasound assessment is easy, requiring little specialized equipment and is non-invasive with no ionizing radiation, yet it provides a more thorough assessment of the lower urinary tract.

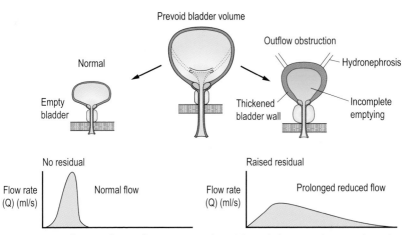

Figure 3.6 *Ultrasound cystodynamogram. The additional ultrasonic data, on the right showing incomplete emptying, thickened bladder wall and bilateral hydronephrosis associated with chronic poor voiding.*

Method and standardization

Ensure that the patient has a subjectively full bladder before carrying out the study to provide a representative result.

URODYNAMICS IN PRACTICE: ULTRASOUND CYSTODYNAMOGRAM

- The full bladder (>200 ml) is scanned using any form of ultrasound probe allowing adequate visualization of the bladder – patients should be scanned when they feel 'full', so providing an idea of the 'functional' bladder capacity.
- The following are noted:
  - bladder wall thickness
  - bladder volume
  - presence of diverticula
  - distal ureteric anatomy
  - prostatic volume
  - presence of intra-vesical pathology (carcinoma or calculi).
- The patient voids into a flowmeter in private.
- A post-voiding scan is taken as soon after voiding as possible to provide accurate assessment of the true bladder post-void residual volume.
- Interpretation of the flow rate takes account of the artefacts and factors mentioned in the uroflowmetry section of this chapter.

INTRAVENOUS URODYNAMOGRAM

The intravenous urodynamogram (IVUD) combines a conventional intravenous urogram (IVU) with uroflowmetry thus providing markedly more information than either investigation alone.

Indications and aims

This test is of value in patients who are to undergo imaging of the upper urinary tracts using an IVU. The addition of uroflowmetry also provides a comprehensive assessment of the lower urinary tract including an estimation of the pre-void bladder volume and the post-void residual (PVR). It is of particular value because it can be easily integrated into the routine of the radiology department and involves little additional equipment or staff training.

Method and standardization

Ensure that the patient has a subjectively full bladder before carrying out the study, to provide a representative result.

URODYNAMICS IN PRACTICE: INTRAVENOUS URODYNAMOGRAM

- An intravenous urogram (IVU) is performed to assess the upper tracts.
- When the patient feels that his or her bladder is naturally full (an event that can be hastened by using a suitable diuretic), uroflowmetry is performed.
- The subsequent post-micturition film after natural micturition allows accurate assessment of the patient's true bladder residual volume.

URETHRAL PRESSURE MEASUREMENT

Originally urethral pressure measurement and in particular urethral pressure profilometry (UPP) enjoyed a disproportionate amount of attention. However the techniques for the investigation of urethral sphincteric function are far from satisfactory and their clinical utility has been questioned; therefore, most experts consider them as research tools and not suitable for widespread clinical usage.

New developments in technology such as air charged technology with true circumferential recording and ease of recording are leading to a resurgence of interest in urethral pressure measurements and may lead to an increasing understanding of the clinical utility of these tests and the clinical significance of the results. However, at present it must be concluded that these techniques remain research tools and the various techniques need to be standardized before urethral pressure measurements can be recommended in routine practice.

The main concerns with urethral pressure measurements are:

- The results obtained are extremely susceptible to experimental artefacts and the patient's degree of relaxation.
- The studies can be distressingly uncomfortable for patients, especially males.
- The mere act of measuring urethral pressures alters the intraurethral pressure and introduces artefacts.
- At rest the urethra is closed, therefore the urethral pressure and urethral closure pressure are idealized concepts that represent the ability of the urethra to prevent leakage.
- A number of techniques have been developed which do not always yield consistent values. Not only do the values differ with the method of measurement, but there is often lack of consistency within a single technique.
- The techniques as yet cannot definitively differentiate intrinsic sphincteric deficiency (ISD) from other disorders (see Chapter 5).
- The techniques as yet cannot establish the severity of the condition.
- The techniques as yet cannot provide a reliable indicator of surgical success and return to normal function following successful therapy.
- Total profile length is not generally regarded as a useful parameter in UPP.
- The information gained from urethral pressure measurements in the storage phase is of limited value in the assessment of voiding disorders and the voiding UPP is not yet fully developed as a technique.

A detailed discussion of the various techniques is therefore outside the scope of this book; however a summary of the techniques is provided below.

Methods

Point pressure measurement

The intraluminal pressure within the urethra may be measured at a single point over a period of time:

1. **At rest**, with the bladder at a certain volume (storage phase).
2. **During stress**, e.g. coughing/Valsalva.
3. **During voiding** (voiding phase).

Urethral pressure profilometry

The intraluminal pressure can also be measured along the length of the entire urethra to produce a urethral pressure profile (UPP). This is

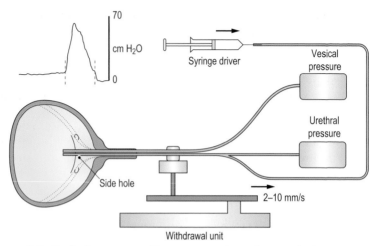

Figure 3.7 *Urethral pressure profilometry,* using the perfusion method.

performed by withdrawing the measuring catheter mechanically at a constant speed (Figure 3.7). The resulting profile indicates the pressures within the urethra from the bladder neck to the meatus. Several techniques have been described including:

- **Resting urethral pressure profile**, with the bladder at rest (storage phase). A low maximum urethral closure pressure (MUCP) on this test may be associated with ISD which may in turn be associated with a poor outcome with certain stress incontinence procedures. The test may also be useful in diagnosing sphincter damage and determining if implantation of an artificial urinary sphincter is appropriate. A high MUCP is associated with Fowler's syndrome in young women with voiding dysfunction, as well as in patients with pelvic pain syndrome.

- **Stress urethral pressure profile**, with increased abdominal pressure, e.g. coughing/Valsalva. In stress incontinence the abdominal pressure transmission, which is thought to keep the normal urethra closed during stress is inadequate; therefore the urethral closure pressure decreases on increased intra-abdominal pressure.

- **Voiding urethral pressure profile** (voiding phase). This technique can be used to determine the pressure and site of urethral obstruction. Accurate interpretation depends upon simultaneous measurement of intra-vesical pressure and measurement of pressure at a precisely localized point in the urethra; this localization may be achieved by a radio-opaque marker on the catheter allowing the pressure measurements to be related to a visualized point in the urethra. Pressures measured whilst voiding are the fluid pressures in the urethra and not the urethral pressure.

Fluid bridge test

A related but different test of bladder neck competence has been described. The test can detect the entry of fluid into the proximal urethra because a continuity of fluid (fluid bridge) between the bladder and urethra occurs in such a situation. The pressure transmission is measured down the infusion channel of a standard Brown–Wickham perfusion catheter (see below) but with the perfusion switched off.

URODYNAMICS IN PRACTICE – URETHRAL PRESSURE MEASUREMENT TECHNIQUES

Perfusion method
- The perfusion method first described by Brown and Wickham is most widely used and is the measurement of the pressure needed to perfuse a catheter at a constant rate (Figure 3.7).
- The catheter has a dual lumen; one for pressure measurements opening at the end of the catheter and the other for perfusion via two opposing side holes 5 cm from the tip of the catheter.
- The catheter is constantly perfused at a set rate using a syringe pump (2–10 ml/min) while being withdrawn at a speed of less than 0.7 ml/s.

Catheter-mounted (microtip) transducers
- These eliminate errors associated with the use of fluid (leaks and air bubbles), but introduce artefacts related to the orientation of the catheter-mounted transducers on the catheter. In addition they do not measure the urethral pressure directly but instead measure the stress imparted by the urethral tissue on the surface of the transducer only.

Balloon catheter profilometry
- Uses a small soft balloon mounted on a catheter.
- Pressure is transmitted by a fluid column to the external pressure transducer.
- Measures urethral pressure accurately, but this technique is the most difficult to use and requires frequent recalibration.

Air charged technology (see Chapter 4)
- Uses a small balloon mounted on a catheter.
- Pressure is transmitted by an air column to the external pressure transducer.
- Measures urethral pressure accurately and easily, and is omni-directional.

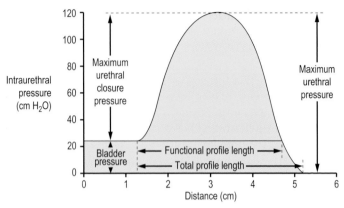

Figure 3.8 *Diagram of a female urethral pressure profile in storage phase* with the nomenclature recommended by the International Continence Society. (Reproduced with permission from Neurourology and Urodynamics 1988; 7:403–426.)

Practical points

When measuring the urethral pressures all systems should be zeroed to atmospheric pressure; the reference point should be taken as the superior edge of the symphysis pubis for external transducers or the transducer itself for catheter-mounted transducers. Intra-vesical pressure should be simultaneously measured to exclude a detrusor contraction and subtraction of the intra-vesical pressure from the urethral pressure produces the urethral closure pressure profile.

The following information is essential when reporting and interpreting the results of urethral pressure studies:

- bladder fullness
- position of patient, as posture affects the urethral muscle tone
- measurement technique
- size and type of catheter
- rate of infusion (perfusion method)
- infusion medium (liquid or gas)
- stationary, continuous, or intermittent withdrawal of catheter
- rate of withdrawal
- orientation of the sensor (catheter transducers)
- period of time of recording
- manoeuvres, e.g. cough and Valsalva.

Urodynamic parameters measured by urethral profilometry

TERMINOLOGY: URETHRAL PRESSURE PROFILES (Figure 3.8)

Urethral pressure: The fluid pressure needed to just open a closed urethra.

The urethral pressure profile: Graph indicating the intraluminal pressure along the length of the urethra.

The urethral closure pressure profile: Derived by the subtraction of intra-vesical pressure from urethral pressure.

Maximum urethral pressure: The maximum pressure of the measured profile.

Maximum urethral closure pressure (MUCP): The maximum difference between the urethral pressure and the intra-vesical pressure.

It is thought that a low MUCP (<20 cm H_2O) may be associated with intrinsic sphincter deficiency (ISD), whereas a high MUCP may suggest bladder neck hypermobility. However the literature on this subject is contradictory, reflecting both the variability in techniques used and inconsistency of results.

Functional profile length: The length of the urethra along which the urethral pressure exceeds intra-vesical pressure.

Pressure 'transmission' ratio: The increment in urethral pressure on stress as a percentage of the simultaneously recorded increment in intra-vesical pressure (Figure 3.9).

NEUROPHYSIOLOGICAL INVESTIGATION

As with urethral pressure measurements, neurophysiological urodynamic investigations have failed to achieve widespread clinical usage. Neuro-physiological testing allows the researcher to develop a greater under-standing of lower urinary tract function but it is uncertain what added value they provide to a clinician. A particular concern is that these tests tend to only be abnormal in the presence of a clinically detectable neuro-logical condition; therefore there is very little additional new information provided by such testing that cannot be obtained by conventional pres-sure/flow urodynamics and a thorough neurological assessment.

Methods

A number of different neurophysiological methods have been described including:

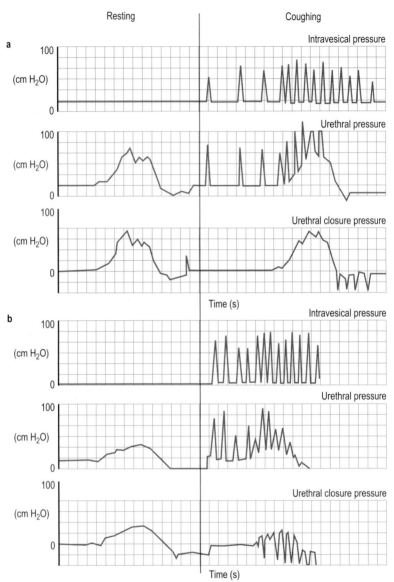

Figure 3.9 *Pressure 'transmission' ratio.* *(a) Urethral pressure profiles in a normal female at rest (on the left) and while coughing (on the right). During coughing there is transmission of intra-abdominal pressure (represented by the bladder trace) to the urethra in all except the distal portion of the profile. (b) Urethral pressure profiles in a patient who has urodynamic stress incontinence at rest (on the left) and while coughing (on the right). At rest the bladder pressure trace is flattened compared with normal and during coughing there is a lack of the normal transmission of intra-abdominal pressure to the urethra, resulting in negative deflections in the urethral closure pressure trace. This abnormal response results from a prolapse of the urethra within a cystourethrocoele. (Reproduced from Abrams P, Feneley R, and Torrens M, Urodynamics. Berlin: Springer; 1983.)*

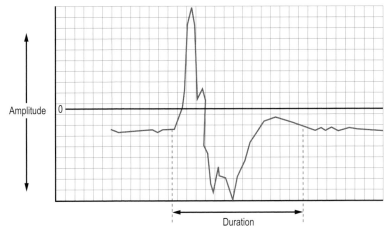

Figure 3.10 *Muscle action potential from a urethral sphincter electromyogram.*

- **Electromyography** – used to study the electrical potentials generated by the depolarization of muscle (Figure 3.10). The action potentials can be detected by either needle electrodes placed into the muscle mass or by surface electrodes. The results are usually displayed on an oscilloscope screen and this procedure can be done either solitarily or as part of an urodynamic investigation. Potential sampling sites include the intrinsic striated muscle of the urethra, the periurethral striated muscle, bulbocavernosus muscle, external anal sphincter and pubococcygeus muscle. Normal motor units have a characteristic waveform which can be altered by disease. In addition during normal voiding there should be no sphincter activity. Increased sphincter activity during voiding in association with increased detrusor pressures and flow changes is characteristic of detrusor sphincter dyssynergia (DSD – see Chapters 6 and 9). This form of neurophysiological testing may also be of utility in detecting Fowler's syndrome in young females with voiding dysfunction, who have been found to display peculiar sphincter activity during voiding.

- **Nerve conduction latency studies** – are used to determine the time taken for a response (latency) to occur in a muscle following stimulation of a peripheral nerve.

- **Reflex latencies** – are similar to nerve conduction studies but instead assess the latency response of reflex arcs which are composed of both an afferent and efferent limb and a synaptic region within the central nervous system (CNS). This is performed by stimulation of a sensory

47

field and recording the reflex muscle contraction. The reflex latency expresses the nerve conduction velocity in both limbs of the reflex arc and also the integrity of the CNS synapse. A prolonged reflex latency therefore may be due to slowed conduction in any of these components of the reflex arc.

- **Sensory testing** – sensory function in the lower urinary tract can also be assessed by semi-objective tests that rely upon the measurement of urethral or vesical sensory thresholds to a standard applied stimulus such as a known electrical current. The vesical/urethral sensory thresholds are the least current that consistently produces a sensation perceived by the subject during stimulation at the site under investigation.

UPPER URINARY TRACT URODYNAMICS

The upper urinary tract is a highly distensible system that is normally protected from the intermittent high pressure generated by the bladder by the competent vesico-ureteric junctions.

The following occurs in the upper tracts under normal circumstances:
- Urine accumulates in the renal pelvis at a resting pressure of less than 5 cm H_2O.
- The pelvic pressure rises to 10 cm H_2O on distension.
- Urine enters the ureter to be transported as a bolus to the bladder by ureteric peristalsis at intra-bolus pressures of 20–60 cm H_2O. Efficient peristalsis is dependent upon apposition of the ureteric walls. Ureteric dilatation (whether obstructive or not) and disorders of ureteric wall mobility, interfere with this process.

The normal response of the upper urinary tract to obstruction at or above the vesico-ureteric junction is to increase the rate of ureteric and pelvic peristalsis; however if the obstruction remains unresolved, ureteric dilatation may occur.

Ureteric dilatation causes uncoordinated peristalsis and inefficient urine transport. As flow is reduced down the ureter, pressure rises are transmitted:
- first to the renal collecting ducts
- then along the renal tubules to the glomeruli.

If there is no parallel increase in the glomerular hydrostatic pressure, filtration will eventually decrease and renal function will become impaired.

The Whitaker test

The Whitaker test is an upper tract urodynamic study combined with antegrade pyelography (Figure 3.11). The principal indication for the investigation is to determine if upper urinary tract obstruction exists, as a dilated upper tract neither confirms nor excludes obstruction.

The principle of the test is to perfuse the upper tract with a constant flow of contrast in an antegrade manner whilst simultaneously measuring renal pelvic and intra-vesical pressures. The test will differentiate patients with continuing obstruction from those with upper tract dilation secondary to permanent alterations in the musculature/tissues of the upper tract. It may also be of utility in evaluating patients with questionable ureteropelvic or vesico-ureteric junction obstruction or those with primary defects of the ureteric musculature (e.g. prune-belly syndrome).

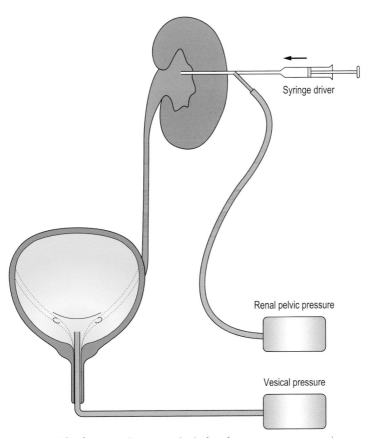

Syringe driver

Renal pelvic pressure

Vesical pressure

Figure 3.11 Whitaker test. *Showing method of performing upper tract urodynamics.*

Urodynamics in practice: The Whitaker test

- Performed under local anaesthesia following premedication with diazepam unless the patient has an indwelling nephrostomy catheter.
- Bladder pressure is measured via a urethral catheter connected to a transducer.
- Renal pelvic pressure can be measured through a nephrostomy tube or through a needle placed in the collecting system at antegrade pyelography – the puncture technique must be good because any leak from the collecting system degrades the information provided by pressure studies.
- Dilute contrast is infused through one arm of a 'Y' connector at an initial rate of 10 ml/min while the other arm of the 'Y' is connected to a pressure transducer recording renal pelvic pressure in response to perfusion (Figure 3.11) – perfusion at 10 ml/min is considerably in excess of physiological rates and should stress the upper urinary tract. However at this high flow rate the normal renal pelvis and ureters will tolerate this flow easily with minimal rise in pressure.
- Bladder pressure is continuously recorded and the subtracted pressure (pelvic pressure – bladder pressure) is automatically calculated – appropriate equipment is available in any department performing lower urinary tract urodynamics.
- Simultaneous fluoroscopy defines the anatomy of the upper tract and spot films can be taken.

Practical points

Upper urinary tract urodynamics is an invasive procedure because a percutaneous nephrostomy tract is required and so it should be reserved for cases where other investigations such as excretory urography and isotope renography have produced equivocal results. The main value of the Whitaker test is in providing an accurate objective assessment of obstruction to renal drainage. Significant rises in pressure are indicative of obstruction whereas free drainage of contrast at low pressure excludes obstruction.

Using this technique a pressure difference between the upper and lower urinary tract of:

- Less than 15 cm H_2O excludes obstruction.
- More than 22 cm H_2O, confirms obstruction.
- Between 15 and 22 cm H_2O lies in the equivocal range.

- If bladder and pelvic pressure increase equally together, then vesico-ureteric reflux has occurred.

An additional indication is in patients with urinary diversion (e.g. an ileal loop). Loin pain can occur because of the high pressures generated by bowel peristalsis causing reflux up the re-implanted ureters; the extent of this can be easily assessed by upper urinary tract urodynamics.

CHAPTER 4

Pressure/flow cystometry

INTRODUCTION

In the previous chapter a number of urodynamic techniques were introduced including commonly performed and important techniques such as voiding diaries, uroflowmetry and pad testing. However, the term 'urodynamics' is usually (incorrectly) used to solely describe the technique of pressure/flow cystometry.

In this chapter pressure/flow cystometry techniques will be discussed in detail. Emphasis will be placed on correctly setting up the equipment according to International Continence Society (ICS) guidelines, correct terminology, indications for performing the procedures as well as how to interpret the results. Subsequent chapters will discuss common lower urinary tract disorders and associated urodynamic findings in greater detail.

AIMS OF PRESSURE/FLOW CYSTOMETRY

Cystometry is necessary for equivocal or more complex cases; the principal advantage of pressure/flow studies over other urodynamic techniques such as uroflowmetry is that the simultaneous measurement of bladder pressure and voiding function allows the site of dysfunction to be localized specifically to either the bladder or the bladder outlet/urethra. In addition cystometry provides much useful information regarding the function of the lower urinary tract during both the storage and voiding phases of the bladder cycle and in many instances can provide a definitive pathophysiological diagnosis for the LUTS experienced.

The principal aim is to reproduce the patient's symptoms and to correlate the symptoms with the underlying urodynamic findings. This should allow a specific urodynamic question to be answered regarding some of the following:

- diagnosis
- disease severity
- most significant abnormality
- future management options

- potential post-operative problems
- the results of treatment
- future problems (surveillance) in at risk groups such as patients with neurological dysfunction.

In addition, during cystometry it is possible to define the behaviour of the bladder during both the storage and voiding phases. In the normal situation the bladder fully relaxes during storage and contracts forcefully during voiding. Likewise it should be possible to define the behaviour of the urethra during both phases. Potential combinations of bladder and urethral function are reviewed in Table 4.1.

Pressure/flow studies also help characterize:
- bladder compliance
- bladder sensation
- bladder capacity
- flow rate (with the additional pressure data not available during uroflowmetry alone).

Pressure/flow cystometry techniques

A number of different techniques have been developed to allow the synchronous measurement of bladder pressures and flow rates.

Simple cystometry – In simple cystometry only the intra-vesical (total bladder) pressure is measured. This technique is not accurate because it assumes that the detrusor pressure approximates to the intra-vesical pressure. A significant proportion of the pressure measured in the bladder emanates from intra-abdominal structures and not from the detrusor muscle itself; since the bladder is subject to changes in intra-abdominal pressure as are all intra-abdominal organs. This technique may therefore lead to inaccurate diagnosis and is rarely performed.

Subtraction cystometry – Subtraction cystometry involves measurement of both the intra-vesical and intra-abdominal pressure simultaneously. Real time electronic subtraction of the intra-abdominal pressure from the intravesical pressure enables the detrusor pressure component of the intravesical pressure to be isolated and analysed. During this technique the bladder is artificially filled with fluid to simulate the storage phase. This method allows the accurate determination of detrusor pressure and does not involve any radiation. It is used in urodynamic units worldwide.

Possible detrusor and urethral activity during storage and voiding

	Storage phase				Voiding phase			
	Detrusor		**Urethra**		**Detrusor**		**Urethra**	
	Underactive	Active	Underactive	Active	Underactive	Active	Underactive	Active
	Normal	Abnormal	Abnormal (incompetent)	Normal	Abnormal	Normal	Normal	Abnormal (obstructive)
	Bladder relaxation to allow filling	Detrusor overactivity, often associated with OAB* and urgency incontinence	Associated with stress incontinence	Maintains continence	Hypocontractile or acontractile bladder. Associated with chronic detrusor muscle damage or abnormal neurology	Contraction allows forceful expulsion of urine	Opening of urethra allows voiding with minimal resistance from the urethra	Overactive urethral sphincter may be associated with abnormal neurology. Prostatic BOO** increases outlet resistance

Table 4.1 Possible detrusor and urethral activity during storage and voiding.
*OAB = overactive bladder symptoms.
**BOO = bladder outlet obstruction.

Videocystometrography (VCMG; also known as videocystometry and video urodynamics) – By combining subtraction cystometry with contrast media bladder filling and radiological screening it is possible to visualize the lower urinary tract during the storage and voiding phases. This results in the gold standard urodynamic investigation (Figure 4.1).

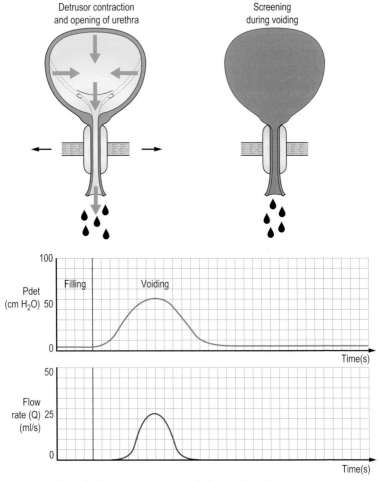

Figure 4.1 *Normal videocystometrogram during voiding.* *The intra-abdominal and intra-vesical pressures are excluded from this trace. The top left schematic shows the detrusor muscle contracting during voiding and the bladder outlet opening. The top right schematic shows the appearances during voiding of the bladder and urethra using radiological screening.*

Radiological screening provides valuable additional anatomical information on:

- the bladder and the urethra
- the presence of vesico-ureteric reflux
- the level of any bladder outlet or urethral obstruction in the lower urinary tract
- the degree of support to the bladder base and the mobility of the urethra.

This information, along with the accompanying pressure/flow traces can be recorded allowing subsequent review and discussion.

Ambulatory urodynamics (AUM) – This is a highly specialized form of subtraction cystometry, which contrary to other pressure/flow cystometry techniques allows the bladder to fill naturally via the kidneys and is performed over a greater length of time. AUM will be discussed further at the end of this chapter.

Risks of pressure/flow studies

The decision to perform an invasive procedure has to balance the possible benefits versus the possible risks and these must be explained to the patient when obtaining informed consent for the procedure.

Risks include:

- Discomfort during the procedure.
- Transient discomfort and dysuria following the procedure.
- Transient bleeding following the procedure.
- Urinary tract infection – occurs in 2–4% of patients. Those at high risk of infection should receive prophylactic antibiotics.
- Radiation exposure during video urodynamics – pregnancy must be excluded in women of child-bearing age.
- Failure – occasionally the urodynamic question is unanswered by the study. This may be due to a failure to reproduce the symptoms, inadequate interpretation or poor technique.

Subtraction cystometry or video urodynamics?

Many urodynamic units do not have the benefit of combined fluoroscopic screening and most patients can be adequately investigated using subtraction cystometry, particularly in the assessment of suspected detrusor overactivity. Suspected stress urinary incontinence is better assessed with video urodynamics, however it can still be evaluated during subtraction cystometry; albeit without radiological visualization of the leakage or an assessment of bladder base support and urethral mobility. Urethral pressure profilometry (Chapter 3) and leak point pressure measurements may provide additional information in stress incontinence when video urodynamics is not available, but their use is not standardized and remains controversial. Suspected BOO can also be diagnosed during subtraction cystometry but the addition of screening allows the level of the obstruction to be determined.

Video urodynamics by providing a combined anatomical and functional evaluation is, however, essential for:

- Thorough assessment of complex cases where equivocal results have been obtained from simpler investigations or previous subtraction cystometry.
- Investigation of patients with known or suspected neurological dysfunction (Chapter 9).
- Situations where there has been an apparent failure of a previous operative procedure.

Terminology of pressure/flow cystometry

Some general terminology related to pressure measurements will be provided in table 4.2 for reference, additional terminology will also be included in the remainder of this chapter.

EQUIPMENT SETUP

The success of any pressure/flow study relies upon meticulous equipment setup and adherence to strict quality control throughout the procedure. The ICS has recommended the use of fluid filled lines and external pressure transducers during cystometry; however if other equipment is to be used then the principles of ensuring accurate pressure measurements specific to that equipment must still be adhered to. In addition it is important that all equipment including transducers, pumps and flowmeters are regularly calibrated as per the manufacturer's specific guidelines for the equipment.

A typical fluid filled lines subtraction cystometry system requires the following components (Figure 4.2):

- Transducers to measure pressures.
- Fluid filled catheters to transmit the intra-vesical and intra-abdominal pressures to the transducers.
- A second intra-vesical catheter to fill the bladder with fluid (or a dual lumen intra-vesical catheter equal to or less than 8 Fr).

Terminology relating to pressure/flow cystometry

Terminology	Definition or urodynamic meaning	Notes
Zero pressure	Should be the surrounding atmospheric pressure	Pressure recorded when the transducer is open to the environment
Reference height (level)	The level at which the transducers should be placed so that all urodynamic pressures have the same hydrostatic component	Taken at the upper edge of the symphysis pubis
Transducer	A device which converts pressure changes into an electrical signal	May be external to the patient or internally placed
Pressure	Force per unit area	Usually measured as cm H_2O during urodynamics
Dampening	A specific type of artefact	Due to poor transmission of pressure to the transducer
Intra-vesical pressure	The pressure within the bladder	Abbreviated to P_{ves}
Intra-abdominal pressure	The pressure surrounding the bladder. Usually measured in the rectum but can also be measured in other sites such as the upper vagina	Abbreviated to P_{abd}
Detrusor pressure	The component of intra-vesical pressure created by forces in the bladder wall (the detrusor muscle) and calculated by subtracting intra-abdominal pressure from intra-vesical pressure	Abbreviated to P_{det} ($P_{det} = P_{ves} - P_{abd}$)

Table 4.2 *Terminology relating to pressure/flow cystometry.*

- An infusion pump connected to the filling line, usually works via the peristaltic principle.
- A flowmeter to measure the flow rate.
- A computer station with appropriate connections to control the pump infusion rate. It should also record the measured pressures and flow rate; and calculate the subtracted 'detrusor' pressure.

It is essential that both the urodynamacist and also the person setting up the equipment and preparing the patient (if different) are familiar with the setup and able to identify and correct any problems that may occur during the course of an investigation.

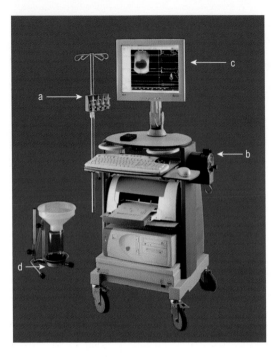

Figure 4.2 Typical pressure flow workstation. *Comprising: (a) transducers on adjustable height stand; (b) pump for bladder filling; (c) display, in this case with superimposed screening image; (d) uroflowmeter for use during the voiding phase of the study.*

Measuring the pressures

Catheter placement

Intra-vesical – During cystometry the total bladder (intra-vesical) pressure is measured by inserting a catheter into the bladder. The catheter is usually passed via the urethra using lubricant or anaesthetic gel. In certain circumstances the catheter can be inserted via the suprapubic route. It should be ensured that the catheter is fixed securely and is in no danger of falling out. If taped to the skin, the fixation should be as near to the meatus as possible; and in men there should be no obstruction to the urethra on the under surface of the penis.

Intra-abdominal – The intra-abdominal pressure is also measured so that a detrusor pressure can be calculated using a computer. The measured intra-vesical pressure is composed of two components: the pressure created by the detrusor muscle, and also the pressure transmitted to the bladder from the external intra-abdominal pressure. By subtracting the intra-abdominal pressure from the intra-vesical pressure the pressure generated intrinsically within the bladder, i.e. from the detrusor muscle, is isolated. By and large the detrusor pressure is of greatest interest to the urodynamacist. The intra-abdominal pressure is usually measured by inserting a catheter into the rectum; however insertion into the upper vagina or into a stoma is also possible. The catheter usually has a flaccid, air-free balloon on the rectal end. The purpose of the balloon is to maintain a small fluid volume at the catheter opening and to avoid faecal blockage. The balloon should only be filled to 10–20% of its unstretched capacity and overfilling is a common mistake causing misleading measurements; often a slit is cut in the balloon to prevent overfilling and a tamponade effect. The rectal catheter should be inserted 10 cm above the anal verge using lubricant and taped securely as close to the anal verge as possible.

Transducers

Three types of transducer systems are in common usage.

External fluid charged pressure transducers – The ICS currently recommends use of external fluid pressure transducers due to their accuracy and inherent characteristics allowing easier use with regard to zero pressure and reference height (Figure 4.3). Urodynamics was originally developed using water filled systems and standardization has therefore developed from an understanding of the characteristics of fluid filled systems. The transducers are fixed externally on a stand and are connected via fluid filled lines to the pressure recording catheters. Fluid transmits the measured pressures directly to the external transducer and any interruption to the transmission of pressure waves may lead to artefacts. Common artefacts include an air

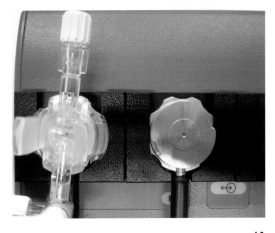

Figure 4.3 External fluid transducers. *Left shown with disposable casing often called the 'dome' which is attached to the fluid containing tubing. Right shows the transducer without a 'dome'.*

bubble anywhere in the tubing between the tip of the catheter and the transducer; air is compressible unlike fluid and therefore a transmitted pressure wave will preferentially compress the air prior to reaching the transducer. The use of some of the pressure in compressing the air will result in a lesser wave being transmitted to the transducer resulting in 'dampening' of the trace (Figure 4.4). This is a common problem and even a miniscule air bubble can cause detectable dampening in the highly sensitive transducers. It can usually be rectified by flushing the air bubble out of the system. A fluid leak or a kink in the tubing will also have similar consequences, so it should be ensured that the system is water tight during the setup procedure and that there are no kinks anywhere along the tubing. Pressure sensing is point sensitive and therefore essentially unidirectional within the fluid filled system, albeit the pressure measurements are not so dependent on the orientation of the catheter within the bladder.

Catheter mounted transducers – These transducers are mounted on the end of special (microtip) catheters. They do not require a fluid filled system and the external proximal end of the catheter is connected directly to the electronic recording system, thus making them simpler to setup than fluid filled systems (Figure 4.5). A reference height does not need to be setup for these systems and they are not affected by movement artefacts. They are therefore advantageous in certain situations such as ambulatory urodynamics, but for conventional cystometry they are not recommended by the ICS. The main disadvantage of this system is that the pressure readings are directional depending on which way the transducer is facing or what the transducer is lying against. Also they do need to be calibrated regularly

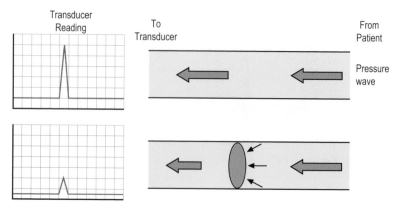

Figure 4.4 Dampening due to air bubble. Upper diagram shows normal pressure transmission. Lower trace shows an air bubble being compressed and therefore 'absorbing' some of the pressure wave leading to reduced transmission and a lower baseline and lower deflection on the trace.

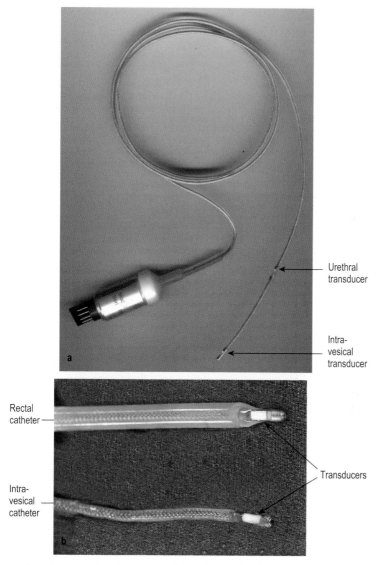

Figure 4.5 (a) Microtip (solid state) catheter. Figure of a dual intra-vesical and urethral measuring microtip catheter with transducer visible distally and further urethral transducer visible a few centimetres more proximal. **(b) Transducers on a microtip (solid state) catheter.** Close-up of distal end of a rectal microtip catheter (top) and an intra-vesical microtip catheter (bottom); with arrows showing the transducers.

63

before use. In addition the catheters are expensive and must be thoroughly cleaned before and after each usage and must be handled with care. Reference height unlike external fluid catheters is at the level of the internal transducer (see later). These catheters should be pre-soaked prior to usage to allow a small amount of water absorption into the coating on the sensing area. Cleaning/disinfecting using a liquid based method immediately prior to usage is sufficient pre-soaking. If not cleaned by a fluid method immediately prior to usage then approximately 20 minutes of pre-soaking is required if the catheter is used regularly; if the catheter has not be used for some weeks then pre-soaking for greater than 1 hour is required.

Air charged, pressure sensing technology – This is the newest transducer system. The system consists of reusable cables with built in transducers, and disposable catheters with a tiny balloon affixed on the distal end of the catheter (Figure 4.6). After the disposable catheter is inserted into the patient and connected to the permanent cable, the transducer is used to 'charge' the catheter by injecting a micro-volume of air into the catheter balloon. This creates a closed, pressure sensing system for accurate, in vivo recording of bladder, abdominal, and urethral pressures. This system is gaining popularity due to its simpler and quicker setup than fluid charged systems. In addition pressure sensing is not unidirectional and the catheters are disposable unlike with microtip catheters. The pressure measurement using the pressure sensing balloons is truly circumferential using this system unlike fluid filled and microtip systems and therefore may be of particular benefit when measuring urethral pressures, as the total pressure generated by the cylindrical urethral wall is measured. In addition these transducers are easily zeroed and similarly to microtip catheters the reference height does not need to be set externally but is taken at the point of the internal balloon. Dampening due to a change in the transmission

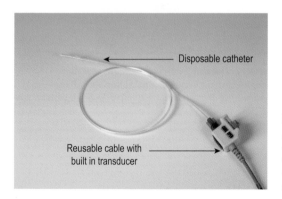

Disposable catheter

Reusable cable with built in transducer

Figure 4.6 *Air charged, pressure sensing technology. A disposable air charged catheter with integral balloon attached to the permanent cable with built in transducer.*

medium (such as occurs when an air bubble is trapped in a fluid filled system) is not a problem in air charged pressure sensing catheters. The pressure measurements are also not influenced by any movements of the catheter, thus decreasing artefacts; this characteristic is ideal for ambulatory urodynamics. This technique does however need to be further studied before it can replace fluid filled catheters as the standard technique.

Filling the bladder

In addition to intra-vesical pressure measuring, the bladder also requires filling with fluid during pressure/flow cystometry (Figure 4.7).

Catheter types

Dual lumen – These are recommended by the ICS, since a single, dual lumen catheter can be used for both the intra-vesical pressure measurement and also for bladder filling (Figure 4.8). The thinnest possible catheter should be used to limit artefacts during voiding due to obstruction of the urethral lumen. However if too thin it may lead to excessive dampening of the

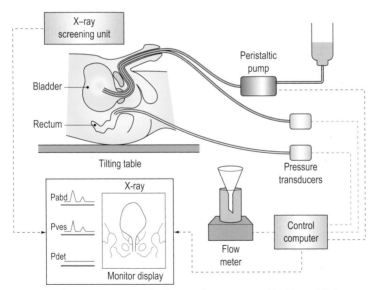

Figure 4.7 *Schematic diagram of video urodynamics. The bladder is filled at a predetermined rate with a radio-opaque contrast medium, with the simultaneous measurement of intra-vesical pressure and intra-abdominal pressure. The subtracted detrusor pressure is calculated automatically and flow is recorded with the flowmeter. This information with accompanying radiographic pictures and a sound track can be recorded allowing subsequent review and analysis.*

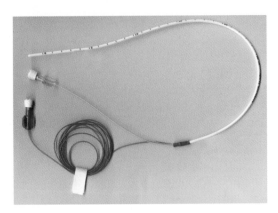

Figure 4.8 *A dual lumen intra-vesical catheter.* Used for both pressure measurement (blue channel) and bladder filling (transparent channel) with a single catheter.

pressure transmission and may also limit the pump rate. The smallest currently available size is 6 Fr, however such a small size is thought to limit the pump rate. In view of this a slightly larger size i.e. 8 Fr is probably preferable.

Single lumen – If used it requires two separate catheters to be inserted into the bladder which is less convenient, but possibly has the advantage that the larger filling tube can be removed prior to voiding. However, this advantage is countered by the need to reinsert the filling line if a second fill/void cycle needs to be performed.

A note should be made of the type, size and number of catheters utilized during an investigation.

Filling fluid
The following can all be used for filling during cystometry:
- sterile water
- normal saline
- radiological contrast – during video urodynamics.

However it is important that the pump and flowmeter are calibrated for the fluid used and it is therefore inadvisable to change the type of filling fluid part way through a study as accurate calibration would not be possible.

Fluid temperature
Ideally the fluid should be at body temperature, however it is more practical to use fluid at room temperature and this does not appear to affect the results. Colder fluids (<14 degrees centigrade) may irritate the bladder and precipitate detrusor overactivity.

Quality control

Once the pressure measuring and filling apparatus are setup it is important to ensure that the pressures are being recorded correctly and rectify any problems prior to commencing the study.

Setting the zero pressure

The pressure measurements can be 'zeroed' either to the surrounding atmospheric pressure or to the internal pressure. However the ICS have recommended that the surrounding atmospheric pressure should be used as it facilitates standardization of the technique and comparison of data to that from other centres.

To zero to atmospheric pressure both the transducer measuring intra-vesical pressure and the transducer measuring intra-abdominal pressure must be opened to the atmosphere. This is easily facilitated if 3-way taps are incorporated into a fluid filled setup (Figure 4.9).

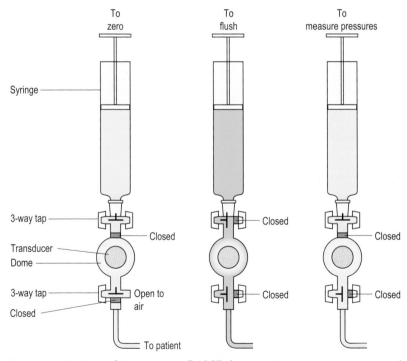

Figure 4.9 Position of 3-way taps in fluid filled system. *Diagram showing position of 3-way taps between transducer and syringe and between transducer and tubing leading to patient. Various positions of the 3-way taps allow the transducer to be zeroed to atmospheric pressure, tubing to be flushed or pressure to be measured.*

67

Setting the reference height

External fluid filled system – The reference height is the level at which the transducers must be placed so that all urodynamic pressures have the same hydrostatic component. To ensure standardization the ICS has defined the reference height as the superior edge of the symphysis pubis. The transducers are usually mounted on an adjustable stand and should be moved so they are level with the symphysis pubis prior to commencing the study (Figure 4.10).

URODYNAMICS IN PRACTICE – REFERENCE HEIGHT

- It is important that the reference height is kept at the level of the symphysis pubis throughout the investigation.
- Therefore, any changes in patient position require the transducer height to be immediately adjusted.
- It is often difficult to maintain the transducers at the level of the symphysis pubis in fluid filled systems when there are rapid movements such as certain provocation tests (heel bouncing, star jumps). In addition, in fluid filled systems rapid movements will result in significant movement artefacts.

Microtip and air filled systems – For microtip transducers the reference height is the transducer itself; for air filled transducers the reference height is at the position of the internal balloon. Using these systems it is therefore difficult to be certain of the position of the reference height or to ensure that the reference height of the intra-abdominal and the intra-vesical lines are equal, unless screening can show the position of the catheters (Figure 4.11). In addition alterations in the position of the patient (i.e. supine to standing) can cause significant differences in the relative positions of the intra-vesical and intra-abdominal transducers/balloons. In the supine position the rectal line is likely to be lower than the intra-vesical line, when standing the rectal line may be higher than the intra-vesical line. In practical terms these differences in height are unlikely to result in a significant effect on results.

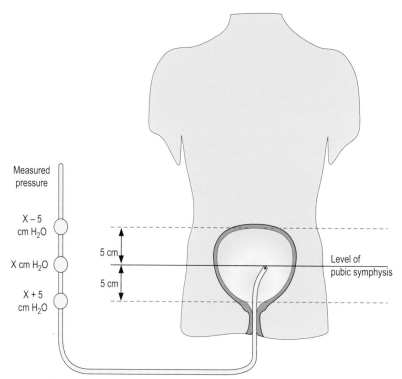

Figure 4.10 *Position of external fluid filled transducers. These should be set at the level of the pubic symphysis to allow standardization and comparison. Increasing the height of the external transducer lowers the measured pressure whereas lowering the height increases the measured pressure. The position of the catheter in the organ has no effect on the measured pressure.*

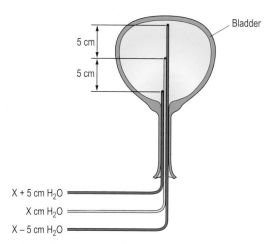

Figure 4.11 *Position of microtip transducer or air filled balloon. The position of the internal transducer or balloon within the bladder alters the measured pressure. If the position is lower, then a higher pressure will be measured due to the extra fluid column above the transducer/balloon: a high position will therefore have a lower pressure.*

Expected resting range of intra-abdominal and intra-vesical pressures

Position	Expected range for intra-abdominal and intra-vesical resting measurements
Supine	5–20 cm H_2O
Sitting	15–40 cm H_2O
Standing	30–50 cm H_2O

Table 4.3 *Expected resting range of intra-abdominal and intra-vesical pressures.*

Resting pressures

Prior to commencing bladder filling it is important to ensure that the initial values are in the expected range (Table 4.3). If the measured pressures lie outside of this range then this suggests a technical problem exists which needs to be rectified. Simple measures such as flushing the lines and checking for fluid leaks and kinks should be performed first.

Due to the pressure subtraction the P_{det} should be <6 cm H_2O and ideally as close to zero as possible.

URODYNAMICS IN PRACTICE – TROUBLESHOOTING RESTING PRESSURES

- If the P_{det} is too high (>6 cm H_2O)
  - The P_{abd} may be too low – the rectal catheter may be kinked/blocked or may contain air bubbles or a fluid leak; therefore flush system, exclude leaks and kinks.
  - The P_{ves} may be too high – the vesical catheter may have been misplaced in the urethral sphincter or the tubing may be kinked; therefore exclude kinks and if necessary adjust position of the catheter.
- If the P_{det} is negative
  - The P_{abd} may be too high – the rectal catheter may have been misplaced, is resting against the rectal wall or the tubing may be kinked; therefore check position and exclude kinks. The rectal balloon may have a tamponade; therefore drain a few drops of fluid from the intra-abdominal measurement system or make a hole in the rectal balloon to remove excess fluid.
  - The P_{ves} may be too low – the vesical catheter may be kinked or may contain air bubbles or a fluid leak; therefore flush system and exclude leaks and kinks.

Dampening and subtraction

Having ensured that the resting values are as expected, any dampening must be identified and rectified. This is performed by asking the patient to cough; both the intra-abdominal and intra-vesical traces should respond equally with a rapid peak and a rapid drop and the detrusor trace should be unaffected. A small biphasic 'blip' is normal in the detrusor trace but any rise/fall in the detrusor pressure during the cough suggests dampening in either the intra-abdominal or the intra-vesical systems (Figure 4.12).

URODYNAMICS IN PRACTICE – ASSESS FOR DAMPENING

- Coughs to assess for dampening should be performed at the beginning and end of the investigation.
- Dampening should be assessed throughout the investigation by having the patient cough every minute (Figure 4.13).
- Coughs should also be performed before and after any major events such as position changes, voids and spontaneous leaks, because catheters may become displaced during these events.
- Any dampening should be immediately corrected.
- Usually the dampening is occurring in the intra-abdominal or intra-vesical line that is deflected the least on coughing.

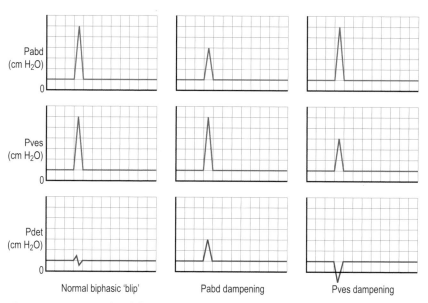

Pabd (cm H$_2$O)

Pves (cm H$_2$O)

Pdet (cm H$_2$O)

Normal biphasic 'blip'   Pabd dampening   Pves dampening

Figure 4.12 *Normal and dampened pressure transmission. Left – good subtraction with no dampening. Middle – intra-abdominal line dampening. Right – intra-vesical line dampening.*

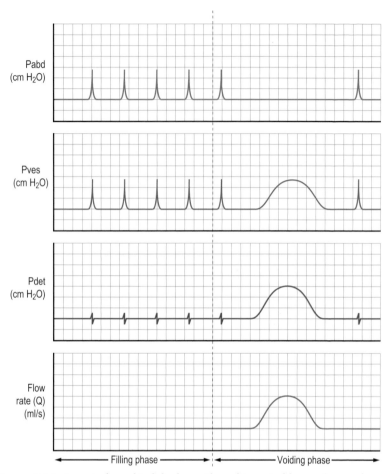

Figure 4.13 *Layout of graphical display, with quality control by regular coughs.* Showing the order of the displayed traces as recommended by the ICS. Subtraction and dampening is assessed every minute by coughs during filling and before and after voiding.

Medications

The patient should not be taking drugs that affect lower urinary tract symptoms, so as to obtain the best indication of the unaltered underlying pathophysiology. The medications should have been discontinued sufficiently prior to the test to allow any effects to have dissipated. We normally suggest discontinuing 1 week prior to the study. Any variations from this ideal must be taken into account when interpreting results and should be clearly recorded.

Sometimes it is beneficial to study patients while taking antimuscarinic agents:

- To evaluate the competence of the outlet in a patient with mixed incontinence and whose detrusor overactivity is controlled with antimuscarinics.
- To reassess detrusor pressure in patients with high pressure neurogenic bladder overactivity treated with antimuscarinics.

PERFORMING PRESSURE/FLOW CYSTOMETRY OR VIDEO CYSTOMETRY

Computer display

The graphical display on the computer monitor ± paper trace will usually have been pre-configured, however these are modifiable and the ICS recommends for consistency that the:

- intra-abdominal pressure (P_{abd}) is displayed at the top
- intra-vesical pressure (P_{ves}) next
- subtracted detrusor pressure (P_{det}) next
- urinary flow rate (Q) is displayed at the bottom (Figure 4.13)
- infused volume, voided volume, urethral pressure, EMG traces and video screening images can be displayed optionally.

Cystometry stages

Pressure/flow cystometry is split into two phases mirroring the normal bladder cycle. The urethral and the detrusor function should be evaluated in both phases.

- Storage/filling phase (also termed as filling cystometry):
  - commences when the pump is turned on
  - ends when the patient and the urodynamacist decide that 'permission to void' has been given (usually at maximum tolerated capacity).
- Voiding phase (also termed as voiding cystometry):
  - commences when the patient and the urodynamicist decide that 'permission to void' has been given, or when uncontrollable voiding begins
  - ends when the patient considers that voiding has finished.

Storage phase

Having made sure that the equipment is setup correctly, working as expected and ensured that the measurements are of good quality, then the pressure/flow cystometry can commence.

Upon starting recording:
- A cough should be performed to record the initial quality of the trace.
- The pump should be commenced at the required fill rate.
- An assessment should be made of the initial residual (see below).

Fill rate

The rate of filling should have been decided prior to beginning the procedure. The ICS originally categorised this into three fill rates:
- **Slow fill:** <10 ml/min) – a more 'physiological' filling rate, used in neurogenic patients.
- **Medium fill:** 10–100 ml/min – the most frequent filling rate.
- **Rapid fill:** >100 ml/min – a very rapid provocative filling rate.

In practice most patients will be filled at a medium fill rate and the ICS has more recently therefore decided to instead categorize fill rates as being either physiological or non-physiological, based on body weight. We would advocate a rate of 50 ml/min in non-neurogenic patients and 20 ml/min in neurogenic patients as being a good balance between performing the investigation rapidly and provoking the detrusor by an abnormally high filling rate. Quality control coughs performed every minute will therefore be every 50 ml filled in non-neurogenic patients.

Patient position

The most physiological position and the position in which most patients experience troublesome symptoms is during standing, and ideally patients should be in the standing position for some part of the filling phase of cystometry. Whilst standing the greatest external pressure is placed on the bladder, and this may be sufficient to provoke detrusor overactivity. In addition many patients only demonstrate stress urinary incontinence when standing. During the voiding phase the patient should be in the position that they usually void (commonly standing for men and sitting for women).

In practice as the catheters are placed whilst supine, it is often helpful to commence filling in this position, as any early problems can be corrected without moving the patient back to a supine position. Following this the patient should be brought to a standing position as soon as possible whilst the bladder capacity is being reached. However, variations in local equipment and screening facilities may require the patient to be filled in the supine or sitting positions. In addition, supine may be the only practical position for filling in certain patients, such as those with neurological dysfunction or very small children. The position should be documented throughout the test and any changes in position will require the external transducer height to be re-adjusted so it remains level with the upper edge of the symphysis pubis.

Initial residual

Prior to catheterizing, the patient is asked to void as completely as possible. Following this, an assessment can be made of the residual volume at the start of the investigation. This can be performed by:

- Ultrasound bladder scan prior to catheterization.
- Draining the urine at the time of catheterization.
- Screening immediately at the start of commencing the pump (video urodynamics):
  - allowing a visual estimation of the bladder volume as the contrast diffuses with the initial residual urine to outline the size of the bladder.
- Calculating the initial residual at the end using the following formula:
  - *initial residual = (volume voided + estimated volume incontinent + final residual) − volume infused*
  - the volume incontinent in practice is difficult to measure and in patients with large residuals is not usually significant.
  - the final residual is measured by draining the bladder via catheter (or by ultrasound bladder scan) at the end of the procedure.

Draining the urine at catheterization is the most direct and accurate method of determining the initial residual and attempts to ensure that the investigation commences on a completely empty bladder. However the removal of a large volume of residual urine may alter detrusor function, especially in neurogenic patients who do not self catheterize and in patients with hydronephrosis secondary to raised detrusor pressures; and may not represent the normal clinical situation. In these instances, the measured maximum cystometric capacity and bladder compliance may be falsely lowered by removal of the initial residual. A similar response is seen if the bladder is filled too rapidly.

Communication

Communication with the patient is often overlooked, yet it is integral to the success of the investigation. Communication should be constant and should commence prior to catheterization with a thorough explanation of the investigation and a review of the current symptoms and recent voiding diary. The investigation is unfamiliar and embarrassing to most patients, and the entire urodynamic team must be sensitive to this and must continually ensure that the patient feels at ease. It is helpful to ascertain if any particular activities (i.e. bending, heel bouncing, hand washing) provoke the symptoms so that these can be integrated into the cystometric assessment. It is essential to relate the urodynamic findings to the patient's symptoms throughout the study, as this is vital to the interpretation of the urodynamic findings.

The patient should be asked to inhibit the desire to void or leak throughout the storage phase, and should be told to immediately disclose any urgency sensations felt or any incontinent episodes during the storage phase. The patient also needs to inform the team if any suprapubic or abdominal pain occurs during filling. Usually if pain is experienced then filling should be discontinued and the voiding phase commenced. Any events need to be recorded on the trace.

It is important that the bladder sensations associated with cystometric filling are recorded and this requires that these are explained fully to the patient and the patient knows to inform the urodynamicist as soon as these sensations occur (see below).

Bladder sensations

These are difficult to evaluate because of their subjective nature; the patient needs to inform the urodynamicist about sensations relating to fullness as soon as they occur and these should be recorded on the trace. Good communication is required to ensure the patient informs the urodynamicist of the sensations experienced without the urodynamicist prompting the patient to the degree that 'words are put in the patient's mouth'.

TERMINOLOGY: BLADDER SENSATIONS (AS DEFINED BY THE ICS)

First sensation of bladder filling: When the patient first becomes aware of the bladder filling.

First desire to void: The feeling that would lead the patient to pass urine at the next convenient moment, but voiding can be delayed if necessary.

Strong desire to void: The persistent desire to void without the fear of leakage.

Maximum cystometric capacity (MCC): In patients with normal sensation this is the volume at which the patient feels he/she can no longer delay micturition.

Urgency: Is a sudden compelling desire to void which is difficult to defer.

Bladder pain: Should not occur during filling; if it occurs the site and character should be specified.

CLINICAL NOTES – BLADDER SENSATION

The overall bladder sensation can be described as being normal, increased or reduced:
- **Reduced** – diminished sensation throughout bladder filling.
- **Normal** – normal occurrence of bladder sensations.
- **Increased** – an early first sensation or an early desire to void and/or an early strong desire to void, which occurs at a low bladder volume and which persists.

Detrusor function during the storage phase

Normal detrusor function – During the storage phase, the bladder should be relaxed and compliant to bladder filling with little or no change in detrusor pressure. Any detrusor activity prior to the voiding phase is therefore abnormal and termed as involuntary detrusor activity.

Detrusor overactivity (DO) – This is characterized by involuntary detrusor contractions (IDCs) during the storage phase. It was previously termed as detrusor instability or detrusor hyper-reflexia (when associated with known neurological disease). The occurrence of associated urgency should be documented on the trace. DO can be:

- **Spontaneous** or **provoked**.
- **Phasic** – having a characteristic waveform of repeated waves of DO.
- **Terminal** – an IDC occurring at cystometric capacity, which cannot be suppressed, and results in incontinence/voiding.
- **Idiopathic** – when there is no defined cause for the overactivity. This is commonly seen associated with the overactive bladder (OAB) syndrome.
- **Neurogenic** – when there is an underlying neurological condition causing the lower urinary tract dysfunction.

URODYNAMICS IN PRACTICE – PROVOCATION MANOEUVRES

- These are techniques used during the storage phase to provoke detrusor overactivity.
- These should be used in patients suspected from their history to have detrusor overactivity who have not demonstrated any IDCs during the storage phase.
- They are therefore usually done towards the end of filling when the patient has reached or is nearly at their maximum cystometric capacity.
- Examples include: bending, changing posture, coughing, jogging on the spot, running water, hand washing, heel bouncing, star jumping, increasing the filling rate, using cooled filling fluid (the latter two examples need a new fill cycle to commence).
- Often determining the most useful provocation manoeuvre follows from asking the patient what provokes their symptoms, and trying to recreate this during the investigation.

If DO is detected then the volume at which the contraction occurred should be recorded as should the rise in amplitude above the baseline (Figure 4.14). The duration of the contraction should also

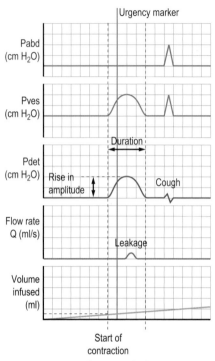

Figure 4.14 *Detrusor overactivity. Volume at which DO commenced, the rise in amplitude and duration, leakage on the uroflowmeter, an urgency marker and a subsequent quality control cough are all shown.*

be noted. It is also important to document if urgency was experienced in association with the IDC; usually a marker can be electronically placed on the trace when urgency occurs. Any associated incontinence should also be documented.

CLINICAL NOTES – TERMINAL DETRUSOR OVERACTIVITY

- Frequently as the patient with detrusor overactivity reaches bladder capacity they have an involuntary detrusor contraction (usually sustained and of high amplitude, compared to previous contractions during the filling phase). Such a terminal contraction is often associated with significant urgency and the patient often becomes increasingly uncomfortable.
- Often in this situation the patient either spontaneously voids or the urodynamicist instructs the patient to void due to the increasing discomfort, resulting in a void 'on top of' an overactive detrusor contraction.
- However when a patient voids during a terminal contraction it is not possible to definitively determine if:

○ the patient has high pressure voiding suggestive of BOO
○ the patient has normal voiding
○ the patient has low pressure voluntary voiding suggestive of detrusor hypo-contractility.

- In this situation it is incorrect to interpret the voiding pressures, as patients may be misdiagnosed, e.g. erroneously diagnosed with obstruction in addition to DO.
- Compounding this, if the trace is read retrospectively and it is unclear at what point the permission to void was given, then the trace can often be interpreted in a variety of ways depending on what point it is assumed that "permission to void" was given.
- Ideally the patient should be refilled and the voiding phase repeated prior to the patient developing a terminal contraction, thus allowing the lower urinary tract function during the voiding phase to be fully appreciated.

Bladder compliance

Bladder compliance describes the intrinsic ability of the bladder to change in volume without a significant alteration in the detrusor pressure. A bladder can either be normally compliant or poorly compliant (hypo-compliant).

$$\text{Compliance (ml/cm } H_2O) = \frac{\text{change in volume } (\Delta V)}{\text{change in detrusor pressure } (\Delta Pdet)}$$

Calculation of compliance requires two standard points to be chosen on the trace. The change in volume and the change in pressure are calculated between these two points allowing the compliance between the two points to be calculated. The ICS have suggested the following two standard points of measurement:

1. At the start of filling: P_{det} usually zero, volume (V) usually zero.
2. At cystometric capacity or immediately before any detrusor contraction that caused significant leakage (and therefore caused the bladder volume to decrease).

The standard points should not be measured at the time of a detrusor contraction as this would give a falsely poor compliance; instead they should be taken at the baseline detrusor pressure at that point.

CLINICAL NOTES – CHECKING BLADDER COMPLIANCE

- Normal compliance is >30–40 ml/cm H_2O.
- Abnormal compliance is <30–40 ml/cm H_2O.
- An abnormally poor compliance is often an artefact of the unnaturally high filling rates that are used during cystometry (excluding ambulatory urodynamics).
- If compliance is seemingly poor it is often useful to slow the fill rate:
  - if compliance improves at the slower rate then an artefact was present and filling should continue at the slower rate (Figure 4.15)
  - if compliance remains poor then true hypo-compliance is present.

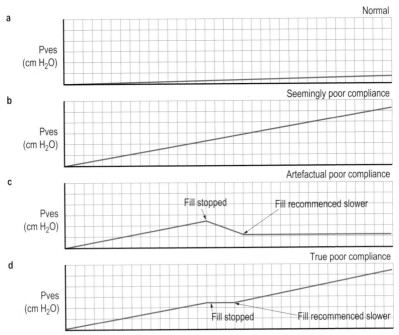

Figure 4.15 *Bladder compliance.* (*a*) *Normal compliance with each 30–40 ml increase in bladder volume causing a less than 1 cm H_2O increase in pressure.* (*b*) *Seemingly poor compliance.* (*c*) *Artefactual poor compliance due to high fill rate; when filling stopped pressure decreases and when recommenced at lower rate the compliance is seen to be normal. At the end of filling it is recommended to wait approximately 30 seconds before recording the end filling pressure.* (*d*) *True poor compliance: stopping filling does not cause a drop in pressure and filling further at any fill rate continues to show poor compliance.*

Bladder capacity

Cystometric capacity – This is the bladder volume at the end of the storage phase when 'permission to void' is given and the investigation moves into the voiding phase. This is usually the maximum cystometric capacity (see below), but if it is not the MCC then the cystometric capacity should be further defined with a reason why filling was stopped, i.e. pain, large infused volume or high detrusor end filling pressure.

Maximum cystometric capacity (MCC) – In patients with normal sensations, this is the volume at which the patient feels he/she can no longer delay micturition due to a strong desire to void. Where there is altered or absent sensation the MCC cannot be measured and the cystometric capacity should instead be recorded.

During cystometry, under normal circumstances the bladder should fill to a capacity of approximately 500 ml before there is a strong desire to void. There is probably no benefit in overfilling patients with volumes above 650–700 ml, as little additional information is likely to be obtained.

Urethral function during the storage phase

During storage the urethral closure mechanism should be fully active and competent, thereby preventing incontinence (it cannot be overactive). Clearly the urethral closure mechanism can be poorly functioning and therefore incompetent.

- **Normal** – maintains continence in the presence of increased intra-abdominal pressure. Although it may be overcome during detrusor overactivity leading to incontinence.
- **Incompetent** – allows leakage in the absence of a detrusor contraction.
- **Urodynamic stress incontinence (USI)** – involuntary leakage of urine during increased intra-abdominal pressure, in the absence of a detrusor contraction. (This was previously termed genuine stress incontinence [GSI].)
- **Urethral relaxation incontinence** – leakage due to urethral relaxation in the absence of raised intra-abdominal pressure or detrusor overactivity.

To assess the urethral function the patient can be asked to increase their intra-abdominal pressure (usually by coughing or performing the Valsalva manoeuvre); on video urodynamics the leakage of contrast can be easily seen as any associated hyper-mobility of the bladder. If the patient is

81

positioned over a flowmeter then the leakage may be detected on the flow trace. If urethral function is normal during storage then there should be no leakage of contrast (in the absence of a detrusor contraction).

Leak point pressures

During the storage phase leak point pressures can also be assessed. Two leak point pressures have been defined by the ICS.

Abdominal leak point pressure (ALPP) – This is the intra-vesical pressure at which urine leakage occurs due to increased abdominal pressure in the absence of a detrusor contraction.

The ALPP acts as a measure of the ability of the bladder neck and the urethral sphincter mechanism to resist increases in intra-abdominal pressure. It may have value in determining if intrinsic sphincter deficiency is present, which may lead to stress urinary incontinence. The terms valsalva leak point pressure (VLPP) and cough leak point pressure (CLPP) are sometimes used to describe the methods of increasing the intra-abdominal pressure. A CLPP is thought to be the most clinically relevant but it is difficult to measure due to the rapidity of the event. A VLPP is slower and therefore easier to perform but is not as clinically relevant, as it is difficult to instruct patients to carry this out in a reproducible fashion.

Detrusor leak point pressure (DLPP) – This is the lowest detrusor pressure at which urine leakage occurs in the absence of either a detrusor contraction or increased abdominal pressure.

The DLPP is used frequently to predict upper tract dysfunction in patients with neurological conditions associated with reduced bladder compliance and poor voiding. It measures the capacity of the bladder neck and urethral sphincter mechanism to resist increased pressure. A high detrusor pressure and high DLPP may be dangerous to the upper urinary tract. Although defined as being measured in the absence of a detrusor contraction many urodynamicists perform the DLPP during an involuntary detrusor contraction. A cutoff of 40 cm H_2O has been suggested as being the threshold for concern regarding potential effects on the upper tracts, but is not an absolute value as lower pressures can also result in upper tract dysfunction.

Unfortunately the methods of performing ALPP and DLPP are not standardized and it is therefore difficult to compare results between centres and assess the clinical relevance of the findings. When recording a leak point pressure a number of variables should be recorded to document the conditions under which the test was performed. These include:

- The site of pressure measurement:
  - ◌ rectal
  - ◌ vaginal
  - ◌ bladder.
- The cause of the increased pressure:
  - ◌ cough
  - ◌ valsalva.
- The bladder capacity at the time of assessing the leak point.
- The baseline pressure used for the test:
  - ◌ the true zero intra-vesical pressure
  - ◌ the value of P_{ves} measured at zero bladder volume
  - ◌ the value of P_{ves} measured immediately before the cough/valsalva manoeuvre (usually at 200 or 300 ml bladder capacity).
- The presence of prolapse.
- The presence of straining (contraction and relaxation of the pelvic floor).
- The method of detecting the leak (screening, artificially coloured urine (dye), changes in electrical conductance, flowmeter, etc).

Video urodynamic screening during the storage phase

Video urodynamics is an excellent method for evaluating the urethral outlet in female patients who have urinary incontinence. When standing partially obliquely the position of the bladder neck at rest and during increased intra-abdominal pressure (coughs, valsalva) can be seen. In addition leakage can be directly visualized and recorded.

Frequently beaking of the bladder neck is encountered during increased intra-abdominal pressure. This is probably a normal finding and is common in continent females. This should be differentiated from the rectangular shaped incompetent bladder neck seen in intrinsic sphincter deficiency (ISD) (see Chapter 5).

In the semilateral/oblique position the bladder neck can be differentiated from a dependent cystocoele and this position also helps in the evaluation of the size and functional significance of a cystocoele.

During storage other abnormalities of the bladder can be visualized including bladder diverticula, fistulae and any vesico-ureteric reflux (particularly if associated with detrusor overactivity) (Figure 4.16).

Voiding phase

The voiding phase of cystometry commences when the patient and the urodynamicist decide that 'permission to void' has been given or when uncontrollable voiding begins. In practice, in patients without any

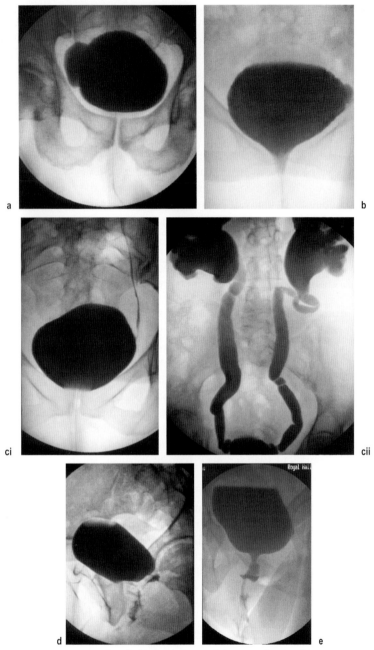

Figure 4.16 Anatomical pathologies discovered during video urodynamics. (a) Large bladder diverticulum. (b) Small bladder diverticulum and stress urinary incontinence. (c) Vesico-ureteric reflux: (i) mild left reflux; (ii) marked bilateral reflux and hydronephrosis. (d) Vesicovaginal fistula. (e) Urethral diverticulum.

neurological dysfunction this occurs when the maximum cystometric capacity (MCC) has been reached.

During this phase the detrusor initially contracts without a change in bladder volume; this is termed 'isovolumetric' contraction. Once the bladder outlet 'opens' and urine begins to be expelled the bladder continues to contract resulting in a decrease in the bladder volume. At the completion of voiding the detrusor relaxes and the urethra/bladder outlet 'closes'. When the patient feels that voiding has ended this phase ends and the storage phase begins again.

During the voiding phase, via the use of a flowmeter connected to the urodynamic equipment, flow rate parameters in addition to pressure data can be obtained and correlated with each other.

Uroflowmetry parameters that can be obtained were described in Chapter 3 and include:

- flow rate (Q)
- maximum flow rate (Q_{max})
- voided volume
- voiding time
- flow time
- average flow rate
- time to maximum flow.

Usually during a pressure/flow study the Q_{max} and voided volume are recorded and an assessment made of the voiding time to determine if the void is prolonged.

Pressure parameters that can be obtained during the voiding phase are applicable to the abdominal, intravesical and detrusor pressure traces (Figure 4.17) and include:

- **Pre-micturition pressure** – the pressure recorded immediately before the initial isovolumetric contraction. The detrusor pre-micturition pressure is probably the most clinically relevant.

- **Opening pressure** – the pressure recorded at the onset of urine flow. The intra-vesical opening pressure is likely to be the most clinically relevant. An adjustment for flow delay must be made for this measurement to be accurate.

- **Opening time** – the time from initial rise in detrusor pressure to onset of flow; this refers to the initial isovolumetric contraction period. An adjustment for flow delay must be made for this measurement to be accurate.

- **Maximum pressure** – the maximum value of the measured pressure, i.e. the peak amplitude of the voiding pressure curve. The maximum

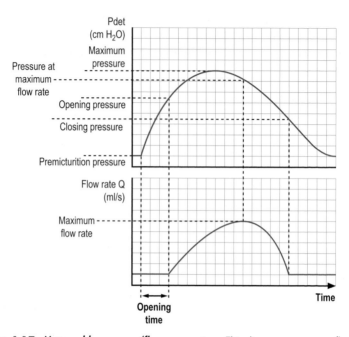

Figure 4.17 Measurable pressure/flow parameters. *This diagram assumes a flow rate delay adjustment has been made prior to correlating the various pressure and flow parameters.*

detrusor pressure (P_{det}max) is clinically relevant in determining the presence of BOO or a poorly contractile detrusor.

- **Pressure at maximum flow** – the pressure recorded at maximum measured flow rate. This is termed the $P_{det}@Q_{max}$ when referring to the detrusor pressure at maximum flow rate. This is also very helpful in determining the presence of BOO or a poorly contractile detrusor muscle. This parameter is used in calculating the bladder outlet obstruction index (BOOI, see Chapter 6). An adjustment for flow delay must be made for this measurement to be accurate.

- **Closing pressure** – the pressure measured at the end of measured flow. The intra-vesical closing pressure is likely to be the most clinically relevant. An adjustment for flow delay must be made for this measurement to be accurate.

- **Minimum voiding pressure** – the minimum pressure during measurable flow but is not necessarily equal to either the opening or closing pressures.

URODYNAMICS IN PRACTICE – FLOW DELAY

- The flow delay is the time delay between a change in bladder pressure and the corresponding change in measured flow rate.
- Pressure measurements are nearly instantaneous.
- However flow measurements encounter a delay from the time the urine leaves the urethral meatus until they are measured by the flowmeter. During this time the urine travels through the air, is collected in the collecting device and is channelled to the flowmeter where the flow rate is measured.
- This delay is variable and is dependent on the equipment being used and how it is set up.
- The delay tends to be longer in men who void whilst standing compared to women who void whilst sitting. This is due to the difference in distance from the urethral meatus to the flowmeter.
- The delay is usually between 0.5 and 1 second, but can be as long as 2 seconds.
- Ideally the delay should be calculated for the equipment in use and a correction made when correlating flow rates to pressure measurements, such as when measuring the $P_{det}@Q_{max}$, opening pressure, closing pressure and opening time.
- To correct for the delay the flow rate trace should be moved to the left by an amount equal to the flow delay. The measured pressures will then correspond with the flow rates achieved by those pressures (Figure 4.18).

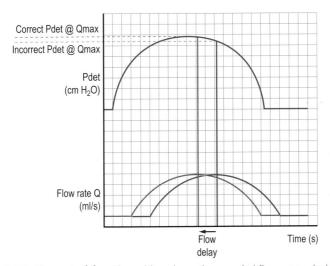

Figure 4.18 *Flow rate delay. The red line shows the recorded flow rate; which must be shifted to the left (blue line) by the amount of the delay, to determine the actual position of the flow trace in relation to the pressure readings.*

Normal values

During voiding the patient's bladder should empty completely with a maximum detrusor pressure of 25–50 cm H_2O.

The maximum urinary flow rate should be:

- over 30–35 ml/s in women
- over 25 ml/s in men under 40 years
- over 15 ml/s in men over 60 years.

Detrusor function during voiding phase

Normal detrusor function – Normal voiding is achieved by a voluntary continuous detrusor contraction which leads to complete emptying of the bladder within an acceptable time span. During the voiding phase high pressures may be encountered with BOO, because the recorded detrusor pressure is not only dependent on the magnitude of the detrusor contraction but also on the degree of outlet resistance. Therefore significant resistance as is seen in BOO may lead to elevated detrusor pressures. In addition the detrusor may compensate for BOO by increasing the magnitude of contraction to expel urine through the increased resistance. Conversely if urethral resistance is low this may be reflected by a low pressure contraction!

Detrusor underactivity – Detrusor underactivity is defined as a contraction of reduced strength and/or duration, resulting in prolonged bladder emptying and/or a failure to achieve complete bladder emptying within a normal time span.

This often results in a post-void residual (PVR) volume remaining in the bladder on the completion of voiding. If during free flow uroflowmetry a PVR is not demonstrated then any raised PVR during the urodynamic assessment can be considered as an artefact due to the artificial circumstances of the test and the presence of an in-situ urethral catheter.

Acontractile detrusor – An acontractile detrusor does not demonstrate any contractile activity during urodynamic assessment. Although one must consider that some patients with a 'bashful' bladder cannot generate a detrusor contraction in the laboratory setting.

After contraction – Occasionally a detrusor contraction which occurs immediately after micturition has ended is encountered on urodynamics. The significance of this finding is unknown and it has been suggested that it may be associated with detrusor overactivity, but this is by no means always the case (Figure 4.19).

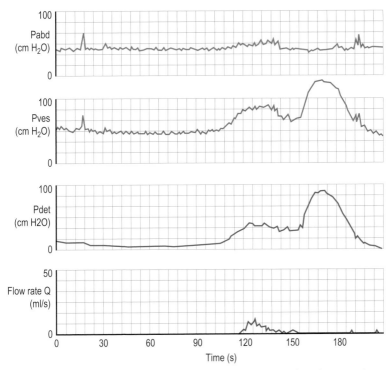

Figure 4.19 *After contraction.* A large after contraction greater than the original voiding contraction is shown on this trace.

Urethral function during voiding phase

Normal urethral function – During the voiding phase the urethra should open and be continuously relaxed to allow the bladder to be emptied at normal intra-vesical pressures. The urethra can therefore not be underactive (incompetent) during voiding, however it may be overactive due to failure to adequately and continuously relax or it may have an anatomical obstruction such as an enlarged prostate or urethral stricture. Pressure/flow studies allow the degree of the overactivity/obstruction to be assessed and with the aid of video urodynamics the precise anatomical location can be determined.

Bladder outlet obstruction – This is a generic term for any obstruction during voiding. It is usually diagnosed by studying synchronous flow rate and detrusor pressure data and is characterized by increased detrusor pressures and reduced flow rates (see Chapter 6).

89

Dysfunctional voiding – This is an intermittent and/or fluctuating flow rate due to involuntary intermittent contractions of the peri-urethral striated muscle during voiding, in neurologically normal patients.

Detrusor sphincter dyssynergia – Occurs when there is a detrusor contraction concurrent with an involuntary contraction of the urethral and/or periurethral striated muscle. This may prevent any expulsion of urine in occasional circumstances. The condition tends to occur in patients with a supra-sacral neurological lesion (see Chapters 6 and 9).

Non-relaxing urethral sphincter obstruction – A non-relaxing, obstructing urethra may result in reduced urine flow and tends to occur in patients with a sacral or infra-sacral neurological lesion, i.e. meningomyelocoele or radical pelvic surgery.

CLINICAL NOTES – THE STOP TEST

- During voiding in a video urodynamic study the male patient can be asked to stop voiding.
- Normally the contrast is "milked back" from the distal sphincter mechanism proximally through the bladder neck into the bladder.
- If there is obstruction at the level of the bladder neck, contrast will be trapped within the prostatic urethra (Figure 4.20).
- This sudden change to an isovolumetric contraction during the stop test leads to a characteristic intra-vesical and detrusor pressure spike (Figure 4.21).

Video urodynamic screening during the voiding phase

Contrast screening during the voiding phase allows the bladder outlet and urethra to be assessed and is particularly useful in men with suspected BOO. The position of the obstruction can often be clearly seen, as can features such as a prostatic indentation at the base of the bladder due to an enlarged prostate. Other abnormalities such as ureteric reflux on voiding and urethral diverticula may also be discovered.

Post-void residual urine

The post-void residual (PVR) is the volume of fluid remaining in the bladder at the end of micturition. Its measurement forms an integral part of the pressure/flow study. However, voiding in unfamiliar surroundings can produce unrepresentative results, as may voiding on demand with a partially filled or overfilled bladder. It must be remembered that the residual volume reflects a relative impairment in detrusor function.

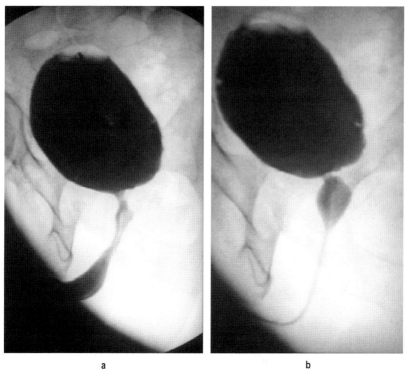

a   b

Figure 4.20 *Abnormal stop test in bladder neck obstruction.* *(a)* *Video urodynamic screening during voiding showing bladder neck obstruction. (b) 'Trapping' of urine within the prostatic urethra due to bladder neck obstruction when patient voluntarily inhibits voiding.*

Important factors in the interpretation of residual volume include:

- The time interval between voiding and residual urine estimation.
- Re-entry of urine into the bladder after micturition; if there is vesico-ureteric reflux then the residual urine may be falsely interpreted.
- Urine in bladder diverticula following micturition; a diverticulum can be regarded as part of the bladder or conversely can be regarded as being outside the functioning bladder when interpreting the PVR.
- An isolated finding of raised PVR requires confirmation before being considered significant.
- The residual volume can be usefully related to the functional bladder capacity estimated from a frequency/volume chart. A ratio of more than 30–40% has been arbitrarily suggested to reflect significance.

The PVR at the end of the study can be measured by draining the bladder via the intra-vesical catheter or, by an ultrasonic 'bladder scan'.

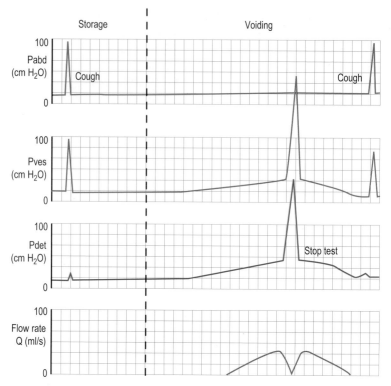

Figure 4.21 *Isometric pressure contraction during stop test.* The detrusor pressure spike during the stop test was thought to be a sign of detrusor power. This is not particularly useful or of diagnostic value.

The PVR can also be roughly estimated (with experience) by screening following voiding during video urodynamics to assess the final volume remaining in the bladder.

Completion of a pressure/flow study

On completion of the voiding phase the patient should perform a further cough to assess the subtraction quality before the recording is terminated. If there are any doubts regarding the quality of the study, presence of artefacts or if a significant problem occurred such as the urethral or rectal catheter falling out during voiding then the study should be repeated. A non-conclusive study may also need repeating.

Immediately following the recording any markers that are required should be placed on the recording. The flow rate delay should be accounted for and any automatically generated values for urodynamic parameters in both the filling and voiding phases should be counterchecked manually. Frequently analysis software mistakes artefacts for clinically relevant data and this counterchecking is therefore imperative to ensure accuracy and any discrepancy should be edited. A print out of the values should be obtained along with the trace to allow for retrospective review.

It is often helpful to record the data obtained on a standard proforma and this can be useful when interpreting the results and writing the study report (Figure 4.22). The study report should be comprehensive and should state if the patient's symptoms were reproduced during the study. It should also answer the clinical questions that led to the test being performed, and the activity of both the bladder and urethra where appropriate during both the storage and the voiding phases should be stated. If more than one abnormality is discovered during the study then the most clinically significant abnormality should be stated; this may require further discussion with the patient following the study. Finally, the study report should contain a recommendation for further investigations or treatment if appropriate.

How to interpret the trace

In addition to calculating the subtracted detrusor pressure, measurement of both the intra-abdominal and the intra-vesical pressures allows the urodynamicist to easily determine if intra-vesical pressure changes emanate from within or external to the bladder by monitoring all three pressure lines. Three common patterns are encountered (Figure 4.23 and Table 4.4).

Activity external to the bladder

Intra-abdominal activity occurs when the patient coughs, talks, performs valsalva, changes position or performs any other physical activity.

Intra-abdominal activity will cause both the intra-abdominal and the intra-vesical pressures to rise synchronously. There should be no change in the detrusor pressure (if subtraction is adequate).

Activity emanating from the bladder

Detrusor contractions emanating from the bladder and during the filling phase if involuntary are a sign of detrusor overactivity, whilst during voluntary voiding they are uninhibited and therefore normal.

93

Conventional urodynamic report

Patient Details: *Date of study: /   /*

		1	**Fill Number**	2
Filling	Fill rate (ml/min)	☐☐☐		☐☐☐
	Baseline Pdet (cmH$_2$O)	☐☐☐		☐☐☐
	First sensation filling (ml)*	☐☐☐		☐☐☐
	Cystometric capacity (ml)*	☐☐☐		☐☐☐
	Compliance (0=normal; 1=reduced)	☐		☐

Overactivity

	1					2				
Fill (0=nil; 1=phasic; 2=nonphasic)	☐					☐				
Cough	☐					☐				
Posture	☐					☐				
Contraction no.	1	2	3	4	5	1	2	3	4	5
Vol. at contraction										
Max. rise in Pdet										

Pre-micturition pressure (cmH$_2$O)   ☐☐☐   ☐☐☐

*Filling volume (need to add initial residual in formal data recording)

Voiding		1		2
	Opening Pdet (cmH$_2$O)	☐☐☐		☐☐☐
	Pdet.max (cmH$_2$O) (Not Pdet.iso)	☐☐☐		☐☐☐
	Pdet at peak flow (ml/s)	☐☐☐		☐☐☐
	Peak flow rate (ml/s)	☐☐.☐		☐☐.☐
	Pdet.iso (cmH$_2$O)	☐☐☐		☐☐☐
	After contraction (0=no; 1=yes)	☐		☐
	Pdet (cmH$_2$O)	☐☐☐		☐☐☐
	Volume voided (ml)	☐☐☐		☐☐☐
	Residual urine (ml)	☐☐☐		☐☐☐
	Calculated initial residual urine (ml)	☐☐☐		☐☐☐

Video		R	L
	Bladder outline ☐ VUR Grade ☐	☐	☐

1=normal; 2=trabeculated;   Grade as defined by International Reflux Study Group (Grades 1–5)
3=sacculated; 4=multiple diverticula

	Males	Females
Bladder neck	☐	☐

In men: 1=normal opening with void; 2=poor opening
In women: 1=closed; 2=open with fill;
3=open with standing; 4=open with stress

Stop test (M)/Position (F)   ☐   ☐

In men: 1=normal; 2=trapping present; 3=equivocal; 9=not done
In women: 4=well supported; 5=descent on stress; 6=prolapse

Prostatic urethra   ☐ 1=normal opening; 2=attenuated;
                             3=DSD; 4=indeterminate

Anterior urethra   ☐ 1=normal; 2=stricture; 3=unsure

Comments/Report

Figure 4.22 *Example proforma used for recording results of pressure/flow cystometry.*

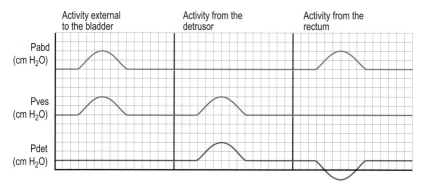

Figure 4.23 Common trace patterns. Diagram showing the three common patterns; activity external to the bladder (intra-abdominal activity), activity emanating from the bladder (detrusor activity) and activity from the rectum.

Interpreting changes in pressure				
	Frequent causes	P_{abd}	P_{ves}	P_{det}
Activity external to the bladder	Cough, Valsalva, movement, talking, etc	Raised	Raised	Unchanged
Activity emanating from the bladder	Detrusor contraction (voluntary or involuntary)	Unchanged	Raised	Raised
Rectal activity	Rectal contraction (voluntary or involuntary)	Raised	Unchanged	Lowered

Table 4.4 Interpreting changes in pressure.

Detrusor activity will cause both the detrusor and the intra-vesical pressures to rise synchronously. There should be no change in the intra-abdominal pressure (if subtraction is adequate).

Rectal activity

During rectal contractions the pressure in the intra-abdominal trace will rise by virtue of the position of the catheter tip in the rectum. However this pressure is not transmitted to the other intra-abdominal organs such as the bladder. Therefore the intra-vesical trace will be unaffected by the rectal contractions. Since during electronic subtraction the detrusor pressure is calculated by subtracting the intra-abdominal pressure from the normally higher intra-vesical pressure, a sudden rise in only the intra-abdominal (rectal) pressure causes an artefactual negative deflection of the detrusor trace which is characteristically a mirror image of the intra-abdominal trace. Repeated rectal contractions can result in a detrusor trace that can easily be mistaken for phasic detrusor overactivity.

URODYNAMICS IN PRACTICE – INTERPRETATION TIPS

- Start by looking at the intra-vesical trace, if a change in pressure is seen then look at the detrusor followed by the intra-abdominal trace.
- If the intra-vesical trace has changed synchronously with the detrusor trace then this is genuine detrusor activity; although double check that the abdominal trace has not changed.
- If instead the intra-abdominal trace has changed synchronously with the intra-vesical trace and there is no change in the detrusor pressure then the activity emanates from outside the bladder and is not due to detrusor activity.
- If however the intra-abdominal pressure is a mirror image of the detrusor trace then rectal contractions are occurring. The detrusor trace is an artefact in this case.
- With experience interpreting these changes becomes second nature. Although frequently interpretation is difficult due to multiple events occurring simultaneously (e.g. a detrusor contraction and abdominal straining).
- Interpretation is also hindered if the subtraction and quality of the recording is poor.

Troubleshooting

Artefacts are common and may lead to errors in the interpretation of results. They should be promptly detected by continually observing the trace and if an artefact is present the study and further bladder filling should be temporarily halted. The cause of the artefact should be determined and the fault should be rectified. Prior to recommencing filling the quality of subtraction should be reassessed with coughing.

Ensuring the resting values are feasible

Please see section earlier in this chapter (page 70) on ensuring that the initial resting values are feasible and troubleshoot as suggested.

Poor subtraction and dampening

A urodynamic study may be difficult to interpret if subtraction is poor due to dampening. The line with the lowest amplitude on coughing is usually the cause of the poor subtraction and should be investigated first. Another clue to the cause of damping is the direction of the deflection of the subtracted detrusor pressure. Normally a cough should produce a small biphasic blip in the detrusor trace; however an obviously positive deflection suggests intra-abdominal line dampening, whereas an obviously negative deflection suggests intra-vesical line dampening (Figure 4.12).

If dampening in a line appears inadequate, flush the line to clear out air bubbles, ensure there is no kinking in the line, check all connections are secure with no fluid leakage and check the position of the line. As a last resort replace the measurement catheter (may be blocked/defective) and if no better a transducer error (rare) should be suspected. After each attempt at remedying the problem, ask the patient to cough to determine if the subtraction has improved.

Negative rectal pressure

A negative rectal pressure adds to the total bladder pressure, and therefore the subtracted detrusor pressure may be higher than the total bladder pressure (Figure 4.24). It is usually prevented by calibrating the lines adequately

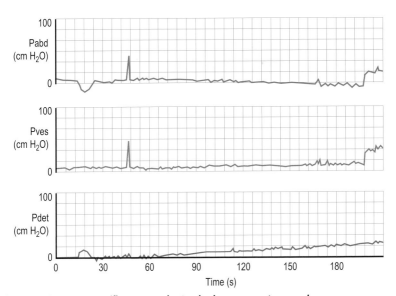

Figure 4.24 *Pressure/flow trace obtained when a negative rectal pressure artefactually adds to the total bladder pressure.* The resulting subtracted detrusor pressure is artefactually higher than the intra-vesical pressure. This is seen at the start of this trace, with the negative rectal deflection curve (mimicking a detrusor contraction) and also gradually as the rectal pressure falls throughout the trace leading to a rising detrusor pressure; this could easily be misinterpreted as poor bladder compliance. The end filling pressure should be interpreted from the intra-vesical pressure line in this case.

at the start of the study and avoiding air bubbles and kinks in the rectal line. In addition when not using a special rectal balloon catheter, a finger cot should be placed around the rectal catheter to prevent blockage of the line by faeculent material and a slit should be cut in the finger cot to prevent tamponade when flushing out the line. The finger cot is easily made by cutting the finger off a surgical glove and attaching this to the distal end of the rectal catheter.

Loss of trace activity

The trace should be 'active', i.e. small second by second variations should be seen. If the line loses this activity and becomes a 'flat line', then there has been a total loss of pressure monitoring, possibly due to a measuring catheter falling out, a loss of pressure signal reaching the transducer, a transducer failure or a loose connection between the transducer and the monitoring computer. The line can easily be checked by asking the patient to cough or to perform a valsalva manoeuvre.

Sudden changes of pressure

Sudden large changes of pressure suggest that either the vesical or the rectal catheters have moved. They may completely fall out causing the pressure reading to dramatically drop or they may move into an area of higher pressure, i.e. the vesical catheter moving from the bladder into the urethral sphincter (Figure 4.25). Misplaced catheters should be promptly moved into the correct location. The catheters may need changing if they fall into a non-sterile area.

AMBULATORY URODYNAMICS

Introduction

Conventional pressure/flow cystometry has a number of shortcomings including:
- non-physiologically high filling rate
- short period of assessment
- mostly performed stationary
- usually performed in an unfamiliar environment for the patient.

It is therefore a 'non-physiological' assessment and may not give an accurate representation of the patient's lower urinary tract function. Detrusor overactivity is detected using a conventional pressure/flow study in

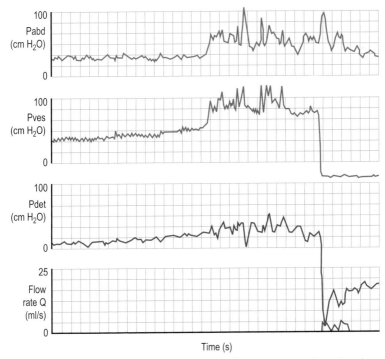

Figure 4.25 *An uninterpretable study due to artefacts.* Prior to voiding when the patient appears to be straining there is poor subtraction and the intra-vesical line appears to be malfunctioning. On commencing voiding the intra-vesical catheter is ejected leading to an abrupt loss in the intra-vesical signal. (Reproduced with permission from WHO 4th International Consultation on BPH.)

only about 50–60% of patients who have LUTS highly suggestive of detrusor overactivity. Despite the shortcomings, conventional pressure/flow studies remain the gold standard investigation of lower urinary tract dysfunction and are performed far more frequently than ambulatory urodynamics (AUM).

AUM overcomes many of these limitations by providing a more 'physiological' assessment of the patient's condition. During AUM the bladder is not artificially filled, but instead is filled by natural urine production from the kidneys. The test is usually done over a much longer period of time than a conventional study, ranging from a couple of hours up to 24 hours in some instances. In addition the patient is able to perform some everyday activities, including actions which may provoke the troublesome symptoms and the patient is free of the fixed urodynamic apparatus of conventional pressure/flow cystometry, with the monitoring taking place outside of the urodynamic laboratory.

Indications

AUM procedures are much more time consuming to perform and require regular monitoring to ensure that the catheters have not become displaced. It remains debatable as to whether they are appropriate for widespread clinical usage. To date the technique has not been standardized and the measurement parameters not adequately defined by the ICS.

The procedure should be reserved for situations where conventional pressure/flow studies have failed to explain or reproduce the symptoms and where further knowledge of the function of the lower urinary tract is likely to aid subsequent management.

Equipment

The basic equipment needed for an AUM study comprises:

- A vesical and a rectal catheter; these tend to be catheter mounted (microtip) transducers, although developments in air charged transducers will allow AUM to be performed with these also.
- A portable storage device to record data (Figure 4.26); this device is connected to the catheters/transducers and records the pressure readings. This device is worn by the patients for the duration of the study. Developments in Bluetooth/wireless technology allow real time monitoring of the pressures via a PC. Most storage devices are battery powered and allow information to be collected for several hours. Extra channels on the devices may also collect measurements of urine loss and urethral pressure.
- A PC for downloading, processing and plotting the data.

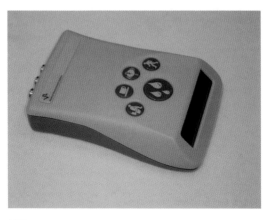

Figure 4.26 A modern Bluetooth portable ambulatory urodynamic device. Can be carried by the patient using a strap. The urodynamic catheters are attached to the connectors on the back of the device (just visible). The device also has event buttons for the patient to use.

- A uroflowmeter which communicates the flow data to either the portable storage device or the PC used for monitoring the study.

Performing an AUM study

AUM assessments should only be performed by those experienced in performing conventional pressure/flow cystometry. Most of the principles of setting up and performing a high quality conventional study are relevant during AUM studies. The transducers should be calibrated before the investigation and should be zeroed to atmospheric pressure.

Often a patient will be left unattended for a considerable length of time during an AUM study; therefore it is imperative that the quality of the pressure recording and the subtraction are stringently assessed at the start, by coughing and/or performing the Valsalva in the supine, sitting and erect positions. All of the catheters should be securely fixed to the patient to limit any danger of becoming displaced during movement. The urodynamicist must be convinced of the quality of measurements before proceeding with the investigation.

Periodically the quality of the measurements should be reassessed during the course of a study and the patient should be asked to cough regularly throughout and prior to terminating the monitoring and also before any voiding episodes; so that on retrospective analysis the quality of the subtraction can be determined.

The procedure for performing an AUM assessment is not standardized and it is therefore important that the method used is stated. Information to be recorded includes:

- Initial residual urine.
- Urine leaked during study – assessed by weighing pads before and after usage throughout the study; or by electronic assessment of leakage, for example by using a conductance channel to determine when leakage occurs.
- The time and volume of voids, including the flow rate will be recorded throughout the study by the use of the flowmeter.
- Length of the study.
- Final residual on study completion.

In addition events should be recorded by the patient, ideally on the portable storage device including:
- initiation of voluntary voids
- cessation of voluntary voids
- episodes of urgency
- episodes of discomfort or pain
- time and type of any specific provocative activities

- time and volume of fluid intake
- episodes of urinary leakage.

Analysis of results

The quality of the trace should be assessed by carefully checking the plausibility of the recordings and the adequacy of the subtraction. A poor quality trace may not be suitable for quantitative analysis, although it may still yield some clinically useful information.

The storage and voiding phases should be identified during the trace and any markers should be correlated to these. Using the same principles used during conventional pressure/flow studies, the function of both the bladder and the urethra/bladder outlet should be determined during both the storage and the voiding phases. In particular troublesome symptoms should be correlated to the recorded findings to try to determine the pathophysiology of the symptoms.

Frequently the results following AUM are different from those obtained during conventional pressure/flow studies. In many cases DO is not identified during conventional studies in patients strongly suspected of DO, yet involuntary detrusor activity (IDA) is picked up on the AUM study. Conversely, many patients not suspected of DO (including asymptomatic volunteers in research studies) display IDA during AUM assessment. The significance of IDA in asymptomatic patients or IDA without associated urgency in symptomatic patients is currently unknown.

The explanation for these apparent differences between AUM and conventional urodynamics may relate to the circumstances associated with the ambulatory test. Artificial filling may be relatively insensitive, being too fast to allow detection of 'normal' or 'physiological' detrusor activity. However, although filling is natural during AUM, it is not physiological to have catheters in situ for protracted periods such as 3–4 hours. Voiding parameters should be more physiological during AUM as less overfilling of the bladder should occur and the results during voiding should be more representative, despite a catheter being in situ during voiding.

Further research is needed to assess the significance of the findings during AUM and to determine the range of normality; therefore AUM should not be used as routine but should be reserved for carefully selected cases only.

CHAPTER 5

Storage disorders and incontinence

INTRODUCTION

Storage disorders are common in both men and women and are often associated with urinary incontinence. Overactive bladder (OAB) syndrome affects approximately 12% of adult males and females in the population and the prevalence increases with age, whilst urinary incontinence affects millions of individuals worldwide, 85% of whom are women. More than one-third of healthy elderly women and approximately 50% of institutionalized females suffer from incontinence with estimates indicating that as many as one in four women experience urinary incontinence during their lifetime.

OAB and particularly urinary incontinence carry a considerable social stigma; many sufferers are unable to continue with their daily activities and many give up their employment. Not only are the symptoms troublesome but they are extremely embarrassing and can have a profound psychological as well as a social, sexual and hygienic impact. Many patients adopt elaborate coping mechanisms including voiding frequently, mapping out the location of toilets, drinking less or wearing dark clothing to mask incontinent episodes. Others resort to wearing incontinence pads or sanitary towels.

However, many successful treatments are available for these conditions; therefore it is important that sufferers are offered a suitable treatment and frequently urodynamics are required to determine the most appropriate management choice. A simple algorithm for the investigation of incontinence is shown in Figure 5.1.

OVERACTIVE BLADDER SYNDROME AND URGENCY INCONTINENCE

Overactive bladder (OAB) syndrome is defined as 'urgency, with or without urgency incontinence, usually with frequency and nocturia'. OAB can only be diagnosed if infection or other obvious pathologies that may cause the symptoms are excluded. OAB is also known as urgency syndrome and urgency/frequency syndrome. These symptom combinations are frequently associated with demonstrable detrusor overactivity (DO) during the filling phase of pressure/flow cystometry.

CLINICAL NOTES: PATIENT EVALUATION OF STORAGE DISORDERS AND INCONTINENCE

History:
- Storage symptoms.
- Factors that induce leakage.
- Pad usage and volume leaked.
- Coping mechanisms.
- Obstetric history.
- Drug therapy including previous treatments.
- Surgical history.

Physical examination:
- A palpable enlargement of the bladder post-void residual (PVR) volume.
- Stress incontinence on coughing (preferably when the bladder is full).
- Pelvic organ prolapse (POP) on coughing/valsalva.
- Urethral mucosal prolapse.
- Introital atrophy.
- Pelvic floor muscle tone.
- Abnormal neurology.

Investigations:
- Urinalysis
- Post-void residual
- Pad testing
- Bladder diary

Must exclude:
- Urinary tract infections (UTI).
- Other significant lower urinary tract abnormalities such as bladder carcinoma or calculi. A urine sample should always be assessed for the presence of haematuria, pyuria or infection.
- Chronic retention with overflow incontinence.

OAB can be further categorized as:
- OAB-dry, where there is no associated urinary incontinence
- OAB-wet, where there is associated urgency urinary incontinence.

It is believed that the driving force within OAB is the symptom of urgency, defined as 'the complaint of a sudden compelling desire to pass urine, which is difficult to deter' (Figure 5.2). Urgency may compel the sufferer to void more frequently than normal and to wake from sleep to void. Increased frequency can also partly be a result of an adaptive or coping mechanism to suppress urgency. If urgency is severe and the patient

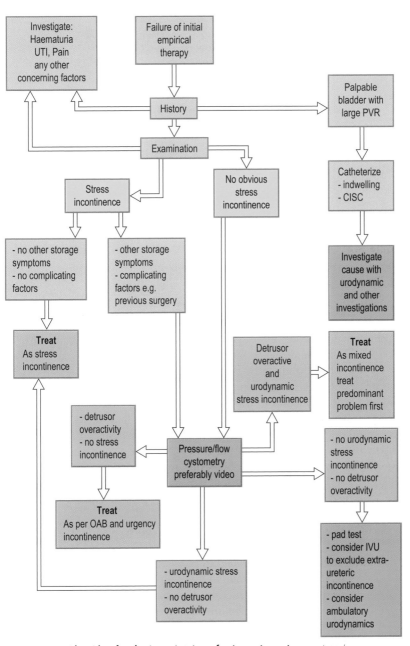

Figure 5.1 *Algorithm for the investigation of urinary incontinence.* Initial
investigations should focus on differentiating between detrusor overactivity and urodynamic
stress incontinence, although the conditions frequently co-exist as mixed incontinence.
CISC, clean intermittent self-catheterization; IVU, intravenous urogram.

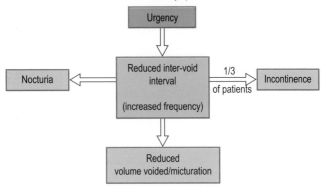

OAB syndrome: A symptomatic sequence

With static intake, urgency episodes reduce the inter-void interval and result in the other symptoms of OAB

Figure 5.2 *Urgency is the pivotal symptom of OAB/.* Urgency drives the other storage symptoms.

has little warning or is not able to reach a toilet in time, then urgency incontinence may occur. Approximately 30% of patients with OAB have urgency incontinence, although the prevalence increases significantly in the elderly with multiple co-morbidities.

As urgency is frequently associated with detrusor overactivity (DO) during cystometry, it had been previously hypothesized that the pathology was due to dysfunction in the efferent motor innervation of the bladder. However, significant emerging evidence suggests that the dysfunction (or its central nervous system interpretation) is at least partly (if not wholly) due to afferent sensory dysfunction and this would be in concordance with the pivotal symptom of urgency being an essentially sensory symptom (Figure 5.3). Though the majority of OAB and urgency incontinence patients are classified as 'idiopathic', a number of clinical causes should be considered:

- Intra-vesical, for instance infection, foreign body, bladder carcinoma.
- Neurogenic disease.
- Bladder outlet obstruction such as BOO in elderly men, urethral valves in boys, bladder neck dyssynergia in young men, pelvic floor dyssynergia and consequent upon obstructing cystourethropexy.
- Iatrogenic, for example following operative treatment of stress incontinence.

Frequently the symptoms are triggered by certain events such as running water, 'key in the door', 'foot on the floor', giggling, exertion or female orgasm.

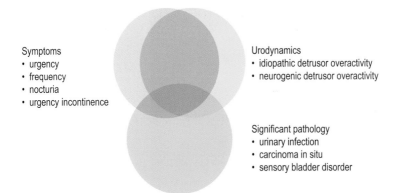

Figure 5.3 Overlap of OAB storage symptoms, urodynamic findings and other pathologies. *Showing a large correlation of symptoms with urodynamic evidence of DO. However a small subset of these patients will also have other significant pathologies.*

Management of OAB and urgency incontinence

A large number of patients are treated empirically often by their primary care physician. If successfully managed and if important pathologies such as bladder carcinoma (Figure 5.4) and UTI have been excluded then there is often little need for further investigations. Frequently however the patient may have equivocal symptoms or the condition may not respond to initial therapy; in such circumstances the patient should be referred to secondary care for a more detailed evaluation and a greater range of management options. Successful management of OAB requires that the condition is accurately diagnosed and differentiated from other lower urinary disorders such as stress incontinence.

Available and emerging treatment choices include:

- **Fluid intake advice** (reduce volume, reduce tea/coffee/alcohol).
- **Bladder training and bladder drill.**
- **Anticholinergic (antimuscarinic) therapy:**
  - Oxybutynin (oral and patches)
  - Tolterodine (oral)
  - Trospium chloride (oral)
  - Solifenacin (oral)
  - Fesoterodine (oral).
  - Propiverine (oral)
  - Darifenacin (oral)
- **Tricyclic antidepressant therapy** (particularly elderly with nocturia):
  - Amitriptyline.

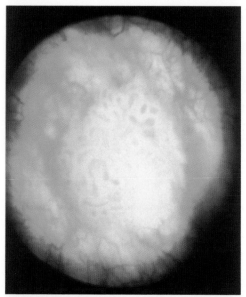

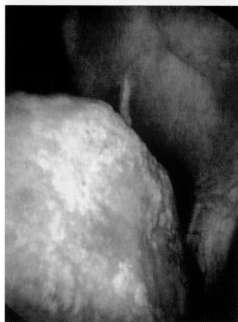

Figure 5.4 *Other causes of storage symptoms.* (a) A superficial transitional cell carcinoma of the bladder in a patient with predominant storage symptoms.
(b) Cystoscopic evidence of a suture and bladder calculus in a patient with storage symptoms following an abdominal hysterectomy.

a

b

- **Synthetic vasopressin analogue** (particularly nocturia and nocturnal enuresis):
  - Desmopressin.
- **Intra-detrusor botulinum toxin injections:**
  - Type A
  - Type B.
- **Neuromodulation:**
  - Sacral neuromodulation (*mechanism unknown but may act to stimulate the Aδ myelinated fibres, especially at the S3 level. Probably enhances sphincter/pelvic tone and may inhibit the detrusor reflex*)
  - Paraurethral stimulation
  - Pudenal nerve stimulation
  - Posterior tibial nerve stimulation.
- **Surgery:**
  - Augmentation entero-cystoplasty
  - Autoaugmentation (detrusor myectomy)
  - Denervation (abandoned)
  - Urinary diversion:
    - ileal or colonic conduit
    - continent diversion
    - suprapubic catheter.

Urodynamics in OAB and urgency incontinence

Voiding diaries – Should be used during the initial evaluation and subsequent monitoring to give an estimate of the frequency and voided volumes. They are also be useful in ruling out suspected nocturnal polyuria. Prior to performing invasive urodynamics a voiding diary will give an estimate of the bladder capacity, and this information should be used to prevent overfilling during the assessment.

1-hour pad test – Useful in patients strongly suspected of urinary incontinence but who have failed to demonstrate any leakage on other investigations such as video urodynamic pressure/flow studies (Figure 5.5). Approximately 30% of patients with urgency incontinence have a normal pressure/flow study. The test also gives a quantification of the degree of incontinence, as patients are usually inaccurate when asked to quantify the leakage.

Uroflowmetry – Not a particularly useful test in this condition, although may be beneficial in ruling out voiding dysfunction as a cause of the storage symptoms, such as in men with mixed LUTS. Should be performed prior to pressure/flow cystometry to give a more representative indication of the voiding pattern than is possible during invasive cystometry.

Pressure/flow cystometry – The gold standard test for detecting detrusor overactivity (DO) which is characterized by involuntary detrusor contractions (IDCs) during the filling phase. DO is thought to be the underlying cause for the symptom of urgency which drives the other symptoms in OAB and which may cause urgency incontinence. Pressure/flow cystometry should be used when a patient has been refractory to empirical therapy, to confirm the presence of DO before proceeding to further treatments. It is essential before considering any invasive treatments such as botulinum toxin therapy or surgery. In addition to clarifying the diagnosis it will help characterize other aspects of lower urinary tract function that may predict problems following an invasive procedure, for example a patient with concurrent voiding dysfunction may be more likely to require clean intermittent self-catheterization (CISC) following botulinum toxin therapy.

Cystometry is also valuable in determining the underlying diagnosis in patients with a mixture of storage and voiding symptoms such as men who may have OAB and also bladder outlet obstruction (BOO). Similarly, in women with a mixture of symptoms suggestive of both urgency incontinence and stress incontinence video cystometry is invaluable in determining if both conditions are present (mixed incontinence) and which is the predominant problem requiring focused treatment. Note that the presence of urgency (but not urgency incontinence) and stress incontinence is known as mixed symptoms.

Non-urodynamic tests – A number of validated questionnaires are available to determine the severity of the condition and the impact on the quality of life. These are useful both in the initial assessment of severity and also to monitor the impact of treatment. Common questionnaires include the King's Health Questionnaire (KHQ), Patients Perception of Bladder Condition (PPBC), the International Consultation on Incontinence Modular Questionnaire (ICIQ) and the Short Form-36 (SF36) questionnaire.

Urodynamic findings in OAB and urgency incontinence (Table 5.1)

Detrusor overactivity

The characteristic finding of DO during pressure/flow cystometry is shown in Figure 5.6. In patients with a known neurological cause for the lower urinary tract dysfunction this is described as neurogenic detrusor overactivity (NDO; see Chapter 9), whereas when the aetiology is unknown it is

Possible findings during urodynamic testing of patients with OAB or urgency incontinence

Voiding diaries	• Increased daytime frequency, usually greater than 8 times daily • Nocturia • Reduced voided volumes with variable amounts • Urgency, if recorded • Incontinence associated with urgency, if present and recorded
1-hour pad test	• Greater than 1.4 g increase in weight
Uroflowmetry	• Possible exaggerated flow rate due to high voiding pressures
Pressure/flow cystometry (Figure 5.5)	• Detrusor overactivity during the filling phase, often associated with urgency and incontinence • Reduced volumes at which first sensation, first desire and strong desire occur • Possible poor compliance • Reduced maximum cystometric capacity • High pre-micturition pressure • Fast opening time • High flow rate with rapid emptying • Time to maximum flow is reduced (often <2 s) • Stop test – the isometric pressure contraction is often high (>50 cm H_2O), rarely possible to perform due to the force of the detrusor contraction • After contraction (unknown significance) • Trabeculation of the bladder and occasionally diverticula during screening (videourodynamics) • Vesico-ureteric reflux in association with high detrusor pressures (both with DO and during voiding) during videourodynamics screening (rare)

Table 5.1 *Possible findings during urodynamic testing of patients with OAB or urgency incontinence.*

described as idiopathic detrusor overactivity (IDO). DO was previously called detrusor instability and NDO was previously called detrusor hyperreflexia.

If DO is detected then it should be ascertained if there is associated urgency and if the urgency sensation is the same as the troublesome symptom the patient normally experiences. The volume at which DO occurs and the rise in amplitude should be documented as described in Chapter 4, as should any associated leakage. It should also be stated if the DO was spontaneous or provoked.

Frequently, phasic (systolic) contraction activity with increasingly frequent and higher amplitude contractions occur as the bladder continues to be filled (Figure 5.7). Often, a large terminal contraction occurs at which

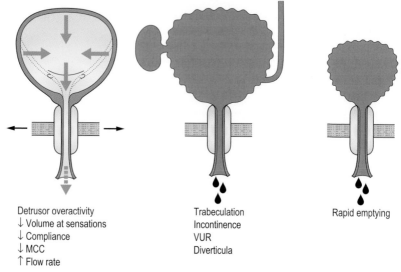

Detrusor overactivity
↓ Volume at sensations
↓ Compliance
↓ MCC
↑ Flow rate

Trabeculation
Incontinence
VUR
Diverticula

Rapid emptying

Figure 5.5 Possible video urodynamic findings during detrusor overactivity. *MCC, maximum cystometric capacity; VUR, vesico-ureteric reflux.*

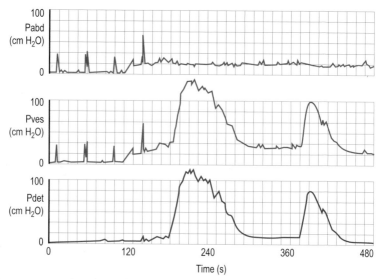

Figure 5.6 High pressure detrusor overactivity. *Note the rise in intra-vesical activity which is mirrored in the detrusor trace. This is the hallmark of detrusor activity, as the lack of activity in the intra-abdominal trace confirms that the activity has emanated from within the bladder.*

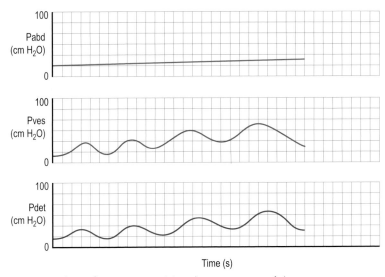

Figure 5.7 *Phasic detrusor overactivity, showing a wave of detrusor contractions, in this case with each contraction rising in amplitude and being of slightly longer duration.*

time the patient feels that he/she can no longer delay micturition and they have therefore reached maximum cystometric capacity (MCC). The patient should be allowed to void voluntarily at this point. If voiding is delayed then the patient will frequently be incontinent (Figure 5.8).

Increasingly forceful detrusor overactivity associated with urgency can cause significant discomfort for the patient and incontinence is embarrassing. Therefore if the presence of detrusor overactivity has answered the 'urodynamic question', there is no need to significantly delay entering the voiding phase of the study as little additional information is likely to be gained.

Cough induced incontinence

Frequently the abrupt change in intra-abdominal pressure during coughing provokes urinary incontinence (Figure 5.9). This is often confused with stress incontinence on the history alone but during video urodynamics DO is seen immediately following a cough with associated urinary leakage. Changing patient position, for instance to the standing position, may similarly trigger DO.

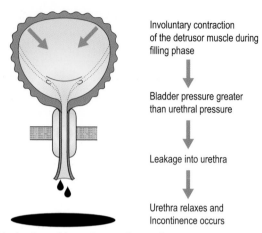

Involuntary contraction
of the detrusor muscle during
filling phase

↓

Bladder pressure greater
than urethral pressure

↓

Leakage into urethra

↓

Urethra relaxes and
Incontinence occurs

Figure 5.8 *Mechanism of incontinence during detrusor overactivity.*

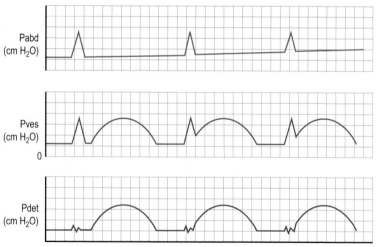

Figure 5.9 *Cough induced detrusor overactivity.* If this is associated with leakage then it must be differentiated from stress urinary incontinence; in both conditions there is leakage associated with coughing.

STRESS INCONTINENCE

Stress incontinence is predominantly a female problem and depending on the definition and the population studied the prevalence of stress urinary incontinence (SUI) is estimated to affect between 4% and 35% of the adult female population, with an apparent increase in prevalence with age. In men, stress incontinence is most commonly seen in patients following a radical prostatectomy.

The current ICS definition of the symptom is 'the complaint of involuntary leakage on effort or exertion, or on sneezing or coughing'. If involuntary leakage is observed during increased abdominal pressure, in the absence of a detrusor contraction during an urodynamic assessment; then the patient is described as having 'urodynamic stress incontinence (USI)'. This term replaces the older term of genuine stress incontinence (GSI).

Stress incontinence can affect females of any age and any parity. Although it is particularly common in multiparous women who have had traumatic or prolonged vaginal deliveries and is usually associated with loss of pelvic floor support and/or damage to the sphincter mechanism. This results in either:
- descent or hyper-mobility of the bladder neck and proximal urethra
- intrinsic sphincter deficiency (ISD).

Many females with SUI will have a combination of both bladder neck descent/hyper-mobility and ISD, but there is some dispute about the relative importance of these in USI and any delineation into these categories may be simplistic and arbitrary and requires further research (see Chapter 2).

Management of stress incontinence

Initial therapy can be commenced empirically by the primary care physician. However if this fails, the patient should be evaluated in secondary care for consideration of a surgical procedure to improve the symptoms.

Available treatment choices include:
- **Fluid intake advice.**
- **Devices:**
  - Pads
  - Adult nappies/diapers
  - Cones
  - Urethral plugs
  - Electrical stimulation.
- **Pelvic floor muscle training (PFMT).**
- **Dual serotonin–noradrenaline reuptake inhibition (SNRI) therapy:**
  - Duloxetine.

115

- **Bulking agents** (*to increase urethral resistance when it is less than that of the intra-vesical pressure at rest*).
- **Surgery:**
  - Colposuspension (to elevate the bladder neck to a position where intra-abdominal pressure transmission is identical to that transmitted to the bladder)
  - Sling procedures (to restore the sub-urethral 'hammock support'):
    - autologous
    - xenograft
    - cadaveric
  - Tape procedures (to restore the sub-urethral 'hammock support'):
    - retro-pubic
    - trans-obturator
  - Artificial urinary sphincter (*can be useful in ISD*).

Urodynamics in stress incontinence

Voiding diaries – Particularly useful in those with mixed symptoms suggestive of stress and urgency incontinence. Useful if leakage (urge versus stress) is recorded to document the frequency of stress incontinence episodes. Prior to performing invasive urodynamics a voiding diary will give an estimate of the bladder capacity, and this information should be used to prevent overfilling during the assessment. Many women with stress urinary incontinence alter their behaviour to try to cope better with the condition; for example they may increase their urinary frequency to maintain an empty or low volume bladder and thereby reduce the frequency or severity of any stress incontinence.

1-hour pad test – Useful in patients strongly suspected of urinary incontinence but who have failed to demonstrate any leakage on other investigations such as video urodynamic studies. The test gives a quantification of the degree of incontinence.

Uroflowmetry – Not a particularly useful test in this condition; although may be beneficial in ruling out any voiding dysfunction which may complicate treatment. Should be performed prior to pressure/flow cystometry to give a more representative indication of the voiding pattern than is possible during invasive cystometry. Exaggerated flow rate or 'fast void' may be seen in patients with significant urethral insufficiency.

Pressure/flow cystometry – Video urodynamics is the gold standard test and allows leakage to be visualized with increases in intra-abdominal pressure. In addition, bladder neck opening and bladder neck descent/

hyper-mobility can also be assessed during screening. In the simplest of cases where there are no uncertainties regarding the diagnosis and no complicating factors, pressure/flow assessment is not required prior to surgery, although this recommendation remains controversial and a diagnosis made on the basis of history alone will not predict detrusor over-activity in up to 25% of cases. In all other cases urodynamics should be performed to confirm the diagnosis, rule out other causes for the incontinence such as urgency incontinence or cough provoked incontinence and assess for possible post-operative complications. For example poor voiding function may suggest a potential need for CISC following an invasive procedure. Cystometry is recommended when considering an invasive procedure in somebody who has previously been treated operatively.

Other urodynamic tests – Electromyography (EMG) measurement during pressure/flow studies may give an indication of the pelvic floor and/or sphincter activity. UPP measurement (Chapter 3) and ALPP (Chapter 4) may help determine if ISD is the cause of the SUI and possibly direct further management. However, all of these tests are non-standardized and currently provide data of uncertain clinical significance (Table 5.2).

Non-urodynamic tests – Cystoscopy adds little to the evaluation of patients who have stress incontinence, but it is occasionally helpful in assessing the short fibrotic 'stove-pipe' urethra sometimes present in patients who have ISD. Complex patients suspected of having a vesical fistula or urethral diverticulum require an appropriate diagnostic workup, including cystoscopy.

Urodynamic findings in stress incontinence

Video urodynamics

Bladder neck descent and hyper-mobility – When the bladder descends due to poor pelvic floor support, increases in intra-abdominal pressure are not transmitted equally to the bladder body and proximal urethra (Figure 5.10, 5.11). Most of the increased pressure is transmitted only to the bladder. This elevates the intra-vesical pressure above the maximum pressure exerted by the urethral sphincter mechanism, resulting in stress incontinence. This is easily visualized with video urodynamics, when standing partially obliquely, the bladder neck position may be abnormally low (below the level of the upper third of the pubic symphysis), signifying loss of pelvic floor support, coughing or valsalva causes the bladder and bladder neck to descend further and leak (Figure 5.12). On termination of the increased intra-abdominal pressure the bladder neck quickly 'springs back' to its original position terminating leakage.

Possible findings during urodynamic testing of patients with stress incontinence	
Voiding diaries	• Episodes of stress incontinence (if recorded) • Frequency as a coping behaviour
1-hour pad test	• Greater than 1.4 g increase in weight
Uroflowmetry	• Possible exaggerated flow rate due to low outlet resistance
Pressure/flow cystometry	• Demonstrable urodynamic stress incontinence • Bladder neck descent and hyper-mobility • Suggest ISD (video urodynamics) • Voiding is usually rapid with a high flow rate (30–60 ml/s) and low voiding pressures, due to reduced outflow resistance (Figure 5.10)
Electromyography	• Possibly demonstrates weakening of the pelvic floor
Urethral pressure profilometry	• Suggest ISD
Abdominal leak point pressures	• Suggest ISD

Table 5.2 *Possible findings during urodynamic testing of patients with stress incontinence.*

Whether to reduce a prolapse during a urodynamic study, both to compensate for the 'kinking'/'obstructive' effect of a cysto-urethrocoele and to replicate the effect of a surgical procedure is often discussed and still remains the subject of debate but limited consensus.

Intrinsic sphincter deficiency – With intrinsic sphincter deficiency (ISD) the sphincter mechanism is weakened and therefore unable to resist the increases in intra-vesical pressure that occur with stress (Table 5.3). When severe, even the slightest increase in pressure (e.g. from minor movement) may cause leakage or the sphincter may be completely open (incompetent) with almost continual leakage. Many patients are unable to interrupt micturition due to weakness of their striated sphincter mechanism. Unfortunately, there is no consensus regarding how best to assess for ISD, with advocates for physical examination (Q tip test), video urodynamics, urethral pressure measurements and abdominal leak point pressure measurements (ALPP > 100 cm H_2O unlikely to be ISD, ALPP < 60 cm H_2O suggestive of ISD). This area needs further research, particularly with recent developments in therapies aimed specifically at treating ISD as opposed to bladder

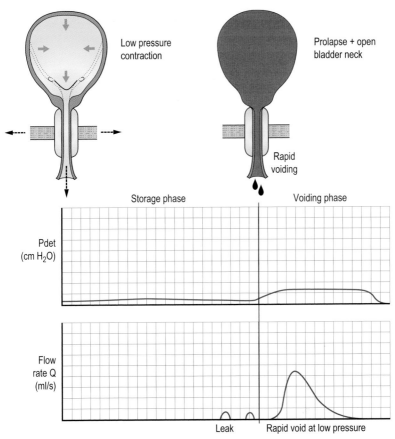

Figure 5.10 *(a) and (b) Typical video urodynamic appearances for urodynamic stress incontinence*, showing low pressure, high flow due to decreased bladder outlet resistance and also showing radiological evidence of an open bladder neck.

neck descent/hyper-mobility. However, in our opinion (based on current evidence) video urodynamics is essential to differentiate between the relative contributions of bladder neck prolapse/hyper-mobility and ISD, because it deals with function, anatomy and dynamics. Typically on video urodynamics patients with pure ISD demonstrate severe leakage with minimal increase in intra-abdominal pressure, there is minimal bladder neck descent and the urethra does not 'spring back', but appears to stay open and continues leaking even after the stress event. Often there is a rectangular shaped incompetent bladder neck (Figure 5.13) and this should be differentiated from the 'beaking' of the bladder neck that is probably a normal finding, even in continent females.

119

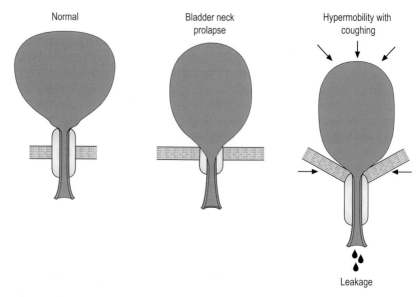

Figure 5.11 *Stress incontinence in bladder neck descent/hyper-mobility*, showing lack of transmission of pressure to the urethra, resulting in leakage.

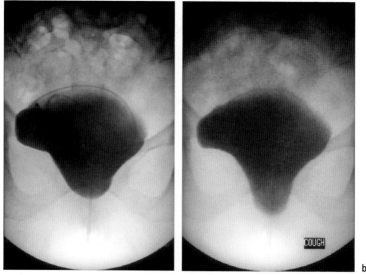

Figure 5.12 *Radiological appearances of bladder neck descent.* (**a**) Cystogram of a female patient in the supine position showing a degree of bladder base prolapse. (**b**) The same patient on coughing showing descent of the bladder base and urethra; on the dynamic screening image leakage was visible.

Contributory causes to intrinsic sphincter deficiency	
Mechanism	Causes
Urethral trauma	Pelvic fracture, traumatic childbirth
Neurological disorder	Myelodysplasia
Vaginal delivery	Pudendal nerve injury
Previous operation	Failed operation for incontinence, urethral dilatation, urethral diverticulectomy, radical prostatectomy

Table 5.3 *Intrinsic sphincter deficiency: contributory causes.*

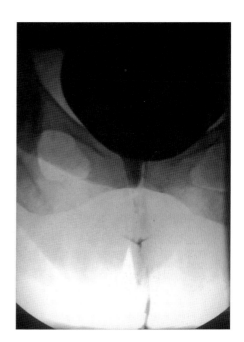

Figure 5.13 *Screening appearances of intrinsic sphincter deficiency.* Cystourethrogram showing typical female patient with intrinsic sphincter deficiency, showing a well supported bladder base with contrast on coughing filling the 'rectangular' urethra, with associated leakage.

OTHER TYPES OF INCONTINENCE

Mixed urinary incontinence – This is the complaint of involuntary leakage associated with urgency and also with exertion, effort, sneezing or coughing. Therefore it is a combination of:
- urgency incontinence
- stress incontinence.

This problem is particularly common and presents a management dilemma, as patients are often refractory to initial treatments and certain treatments may aggravate the other component of the incontinence. For example treating the stress component with an invasive procedure may aggravate the urgency incontinence component. Patients with mixed incontinence symptoms should ideally undergo video urodynamics to determine which component predominates and is associated with the most troublesome symptoms. Treating the most troublesome component first usually achieves the best long term results and often a variety of treatments are needed to optimize management.

Overflow incontinence – This is the involuntary loss of urine associated with overdistension of the bladder secondary to inefficient bladder emptying. It may occur as a result of:
- poor detrusor contractility
- bladder outlet obstruction (BOO)
- a combination of poor detrusor contractility and BOO.

Overflow incontinence is often seen in elderly men with chronic retention. Patients with inefficient bladder emptying and overdistension may present with unconscious dribbling, urinary frequency, urgency or stress urinary incontinence. For this reason determination of the post-void residual urine volume is important in all patients with urinary incontinence to rule out chronic retention.

Unconscious incontinence – This is unperceived involuntary incontinence of urine, neither related to abdominal straining nor associated with urgency. The patient's first sensation is wetness. Its identification is important because it usually represents marked bladder dysfunction.
Most patients who have unconscious incontinence have either:
- significant intrinsic sphincter deficiency
- detrusor overactivity not perceived as urgency because of poor bladder sensation (commonly seen in elderly patients and in those who have neuropathic bladders)
- overflow incontinence (see above).

Situational urinary incontinence – These are types of urinary incontinence that only occur in certain situations, and they may be related to underlying stress incontinence or underlying DO, for example during sexual intercourse or during giggling (often called giggling incontinence); see (Figure 5.14).

Continuous urinary incontinence – This is the complaint of continuous leakage of urine. This may be due to a vesical fistula, for example a vesicovaginal fistula, a congenital abnormality, for example an ectopic ureter, or possibly due to gross intrinsic sphincter deficiency. Some elderly patients with significant urethral insufficiency and/or severe detrusor overactivity report leaking 'all the time'.

Co-existence of different types of incontinence – Any of the types of incontinence described above can exist in combination. As with mixed inconti-

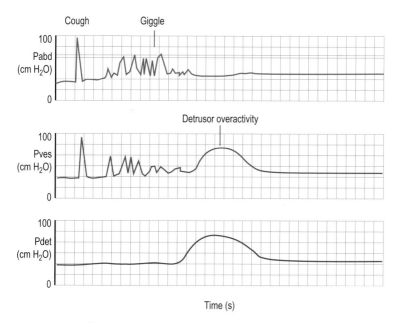

Figure 5.14 *Giggle incontinence. Showing detrusor overactivity provoked by giggling.*

123

nence identification of the various contributory factors are important because they influence treatment selection and help in anticipating post-operative problems. Video urodynamics, in combination with a thorough urological history and physical examination forms the cornerstone of the evaluation of these more complex patients.

INCONTINENCE IN MEN

Urinary incontinence is far less common in men due to the much more adequate urethral/sphincter mechanism. Most cases of male incontinence are due to:

- detrusor overactivity
- neurogenic lower urinary tract dysfunction
- post-prostatectomy (particularly radical prostatectomy)
- overflow incontinence.

Urodynamics forms the cornerstone for evaluating male voiding dysfunction. Indications for pressure/flow cystometry include:

- any type of urinary incontinence
- suspected urethral sphincter insufficiency
- poor voiding function combined with marked storage symptoms
- chronic retention
- recurrent symptoms following surgery
- patients with known or suspected neurological dysfunction of the lower urinary tract
- young patients (<55 years of age)
- storage LUTS refractory to medical therapy.

POST-PROSTATECTOMY INCONTINENCE

Urinary incontinence can be one of the most debilitating and devastating complications following prostatectomy. Its incidence following trans-urethral resection of the prostate (TURP) is less than 1% but following radical prostatectomy for prostatic carcinoma the incidence of severe or total incontinence is approximately 2–12%, with up to 50% of patients complaining of milder stress leakage.

Usually during a prostatectomy the proximal urethral sphincter is ablated, therefore continence is maintained only by the distal urethral sphincter which is composed of both striated and smooth muscle components (see Chapter 2). However if there is pre-existing incompetence of the distal urethral sphincter or if it (or it's innervation) is damaged by surgery then incontinence may occur.

Predisposing causes of distal sphincteric damage before prostatectomy include:

- pelvic trauma
- denervation after radical pelvic surgery
- intervertebral disc disease
- radical radiotherapy.

Sphincteric incompetence resulting from surgery is usually due to:

- neural injury or sphincteric denervation
- peri-urethral fibrosis.

Because the intrinsic smooth muscle of the distal sphincter mechanism is separate from the extrinsic striated muscle of the peri-urethral pelvic floor, most patients with post-prostatectomy incontinence are capable of stopping and starting their urinary stream using the peri-urethral striated muscles.

However, not all post-prostatectomy incontinence is secondary to distal sphincteric incompetence. Other causes include:

- Detrusor overactivity ± poor bladder compliance:
  - Primary – present before the surgery, but only becomes problematic as a consequence of the marked reduction in the integrity of the sphincter mechanisms.
  - Secondary – As a consequence of the surgery.
- Bladder outlet obstruction (BOO) with overflow incontinence:
  - Bladder neck contracture
  - Urethral stricture.

Detrusor overactivity may be present in up to 50% of patients who are incontinent following prostatectomy and may be the underlying cause of the incontinence or a significant contributing factor.

Patient evaluation in post-prostatectomy incontinence

Patients with incontinence following prostatectomy require an in-depth history and physical examination. Most patients give a history of stress incontinence and slow dribbling leakage when standing upright. Many patients are continent when supine and only experience stress or urgency incontinence when changing posture to the standing position. On examination patients who have sphincteric incompetence often leak when asked to perform a valsalva manoeuvre. Any abnormal neurology may suggest an underlying abnormality leading to sphincteric denervation. Overflow

URODYNAMICS IN PRACTICE: POST-PROSTATECTOMY INCONTINENCE

- Pressure/flow cystometry is necessary for evaluating incontinence following prostatectomy.
- Cystometry will help establish a diagnosis of sphincteric incompetence if stress incontinence is present – a low abdominal leak point pressure of less than 60 cm H_2O correlates with sphincteric incompetence, but is not diagnostic. Videourodynamics is particularly helpful.
- Cystometry will identify and characterize any detrusor dysfunction which may be the cause of, or a major contributory factor to the incontinence.
- Commonly post-prostatectomy patients demonstrate detrusor overactivity, bladder hypersensitivity or poor bladder compliance.
- Video urodynamics is particularly useful if there is any obstruction, to identify the level of the obstruction.
- Measurement of the urethral pressure profile (UPP) is of limited value and is generally not recommended.
- The urethral catheter may mask leakage in men with mild stress incontinence; in these cases the catheter should be removed and the abdominal pressure used to assess the valsalva leak point.

incontinence can also be ruled out by suprapubic palpation and measuring a PVR. Urinalysis is necessary to exclude a UTI.

Management

The therapeutic armamentarium for post-prostatectomy incontinence includes:

- Behavioural therapy.
- Pelvic floor exercises.
- Anticholinergic medications (detrusor overactivity that cannot be controlled medically may be a poor prognostic indicator before insertion of an artificial urinary sphincter).
- Peri-urethral injection therapy.
- Artificial urinary sphincter (AUS) implantation.
- Male sling procedures (these cause a persistent relative bladder outlet obstruction and in our view remain investigational at present).

The success rate for peri-urethral injection therapy is less than 30%. The treatment of choice for post-prostatectomy stress incontinence secondary to sphincteric incompetence is the artificial urinary sphincter (AUS); approximately 90% of patients achieve social continence and nearly 50% achieve complete continence. In experienced hands, the AUS gives patients the highest chance of cure and should be offered to appropriate patients.

CHAPTER 6

Voiding disorders and bladder outlet obstruction

INTRODUCTION

Due to the high prevalence of bladder outflow obstruction (BOO) secondary to benign (and malignant) prostatic disease, voiding difficulties are the commonest reason for men to present to a urologist. However, recent evidence shows that a large population of men have a storage disorder such as OAB either as a primary diagnosis or secondary to BOO. Since, voiding disorders frequently are associated with storage LUTS such as nocturia and daytime frequency, this may well lead to a confusing mix of symptoms. With this in mind, men with LUTS should not be assumed to have a voiding disorder/prostatic disease and if there is any doubt as to the diagnosis then pressure/flow cystometry is necessary to differentiate definitively between voiding and storage disorders.

Causes of voiding difficulty in men are:

- **Anatomical outflow obstruction:**
  - obstruction at the level of the prostate (commonest)
  - obstruction at the level of the bladder neck
  - obstruction due to a urethral stricture
  - extrinsic compression of bladder or urethra, e.g. from a tumour.
- **Functional obstruction:**
  - overactivity of the bladder neck/urethral muscles causing dyssynergy with the detrusor contraction.
- **Detrusor muscle failure (poor contractility):**
  - primary
  - secondary to outflow obstruction or a neurogenic disorder.

Voiding difficulty is far less common in females and when it occurs it should be thoroughly investigated with anatomical and functional investigations. Most female patients with voiding difficulty have a neuropathic disorder affecting the bladder, but a functional obstruction of the bladder outlet/urethra or detrusor muscle failure must be excluded. Causes of voiding difficulty in women are:

- **Anatomical outflow obstruction:**
  - ○ overcorrection following cystourethropexy
  - ○ extrinsic compression of bladder/neck urethra, e.g. from a tumour or pelvic organ prolapse (POP)
  - ○ obstruction at the level of the bladder neck
  - ○ urethral stenosis (stricture).
- **Functional obstruction:**
  - ○ overactivity of the bladder neck/urethral muscles causing dyssynergy with the detrusor contraction.
- **Detrusor muscle failure (poor contractility):**
  - ○ primary
  - ○ secondary to outflow obstruction or a neurogenic disorder.
- **Small volume urinary frequency:**
  - ○ many women with bladder overactivity report poor flow, hesitancy, etc. as a result of voiding prematurely at low bladder urine volumes.

ANATOMICAL BLADDER OUTLET OBSTRUCTION

Bladder outflow obstruction (BOO) is a generic term for obstruction during voiding, and is characterized by increased detrusor pressure and reduced urine flow rate. It is usually diagnosed definitively during pressure/flow cystometry although history, physical evaluation and simple urodynamic tests (voiding diaries, uroflowmetry and PVR) often point to the correct diagnosis; the majority of patients do not receive pressure/flow cystometry until initial treatment has failed, or if there are other complicating factors.

Most patients present with predominant voiding LUTS, but some present with complications of the BOO including:
- Acute urinary retention (AUR).
- Chronic urinary retention.
- Renal impairment and hydronephrosis.
- Urinary tract infections (UTIs).
- Bladder calculi.
- Haematuria.
- Secondary detrusor overactivity (*occurs in up to 70% of men with prostatic BOO; it resolves in up to two-thirds of patients following surgical relief of the obstruction, although this suggests a causal relationship between BOO and detrusor overactivity in many patients; recent work has challenged this apparent causal link.*)

Benign prostatic obstruction

TERMINOLOGY: ENLARGEMENT OF THE PROSTATE

Benign prostatic hyperplasia (BPH) A histological diagnosis and present in up to 50% of men over 60 years of age and nearly 88% by 80 years of age – the extent to which prostatic enlargement and symptoms secondary to BPH manifest themselves is variable.

Benign prostatic enlargement (BPE) Prostatic enlargement due to histological BPH. This term should be used when clinically detectable prostatic enlargement is evident, in the absence of a known histological diagnosis of BPH.

Benign prostatic obstruction (BPO) Obstruction to urinary flow demonstrable on pressure/flow cystometry secondary to the prostate gland. This may be due to enlargement of the prostate gland (Figure 6.1a) or to increased prostatic smooth muscle tone causing contraction of the prostate gland around the prostatic urethra (*therefore the prostate does not need to be particularly enlarged to cause obstruction!*).

Treatment options include:
- **Conservative measures:**
  - Fluid intake advice
  - Improve mobility/dexterity/mental state.
- **Phytotherapy** (alternative medications from plant extracts; not recommended by World Health Organization (WHO) consensus).
- **α1-adrenoceptor antagonists:**
  - Alfuzosin
  - Doxazosin
  - Tamsulosin
  - Terazosin.
- **5 Alpha reductase inhibitors:**
  - Finasteride
  - Dutasteride.
- **Combination therapy of α1-adrenoceptor antagonists and 5 alpha reductase inhibitors.**
- **Emerging potential medication choices for male LUTS:**
  - Anticholinergics, alone or in combination with α1-adrenoceptor antagonists
  - Phosphodiesterase type 5 inhibitors, alone or in combination with α1-adrenoceptor antagonists.

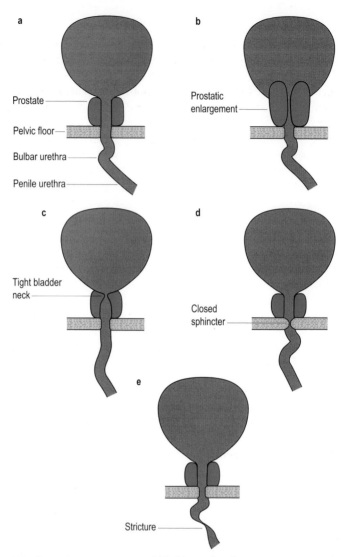

a

Prostate

Pelvic floor

Bulbar urethra

Penile urethra

b

Prostatic
enlargement

c

Tight bladder
neck

d

Closed
sphincter

e

Stricture

Figure 6.1 *Screening appearances of bladder outlet obstruction.* (**A**) *Normal appearance of male lower urinary tract during voiding.* (**B**) *Prostatic obstruction: lengthening and thinning of prostatic urethra, prostatic indentation of the bladder neck.* (**C**) *Bladder neck obstruction: bladder neck shut or narrow during voluntary voiding contraction.* (**D**) *DSD: Narrow membranous urethra, bulging of prostatic urethra.* (**E**) *Urethral stricture.*

- **Invasive treatments:**
  -) *Prostatectomy (usually trans-urethral prostatectomy [TURP]).* Usage has declined in recent years due to the efficacy of medications in reducing symptoms and preventing progression. A variety of methods of performing prostatectomy or ablation of the prostate gland have been described including high intensity ultrasound, microwave thermotherapy, needle ablation, electro-vaporization and laser therapy. Open retropubic prostatectomy is also used in particularly large prostates where the open operation is quicker and safer than TURP. Prostatectomy is more successful in patients with demonstrable BOO on pressure/flow cystometry than in patients without documented obstruction
  -) *Trans-urethral incision of the prostate.* Generally used for smaller prostates, the procedure has less associated morbidity than prostatectomy
  -) *Prostatic stents.* Have been used in elderly men not fit for surgery, who do not wish to be long term catheterized, but stents have a very limited role.

Catheterization to drain the bladder either with an indwelling catheter or CISC may be required in patients who are refractory to conservative or medical treatments and also in those who are not fit or are unwilling to undergo an invasive procedure.

CLINICAL NOTE: BENIGN PROSTATIC DISEASE

- Evaluation of a male patient includes obtaining an appropriate history and, physical examination, in addition to urinalysis, laboratory tests and uroflowmetry.
- Treatment is directed at improving quality of life, relieving BOO and resolving BOO complications.
- Watchful waiting and pharmacotherapy tend to be the choice of therapy for mild to moderate symptoms.
- TURP remains the 'gold standard' technique but there has been a dramatic decline in the number of procedures performed, due to the increasing use of effective medication.

Malignant prostatic obstruction

Benign and malignant prostatic diseases often co-exist, but the relationship appears to be coincidental, although both conditions are under the influence of the male hormone testosterone:

- carcinoma usually originates in the peripheral zone
- benign prostatic enlargement usually originates in the central peri-urethral zone.

Prostatic carcinoma must be ruled out in middle-aged and elderly men who present with storage or voiding LUTS, if carcinoma is discovered then it must be treated appropriately depending on the grade and stage of the disease and the medical condition of the patient, as per relevant guidelines. Initial screening during assessment of LUTS is usually with digital rectal examination (DRE) and serum prostate specific antigen (PSA); followed by trans-rectal ultrasound and prostatic biopsy if there is any suspicion of carcinoma.

Bladder neck obstruction

In this condition the bladder neck does not open completely during voiding and there is little or no flow during a well sustained detrusor contraction. Video urodynamics is necessary in order to make the diagnosis (Figure 6.1c). The condition is especially prevalent in younger men and also occurs occasionally in women; currently the aetiology of primary bladder neck obstruction is unknown. Theories for the cause include fibrosis, neurogenic dysfunction (detrusor/bladder neck dyssynergia) and smooth muscle hypertrophy, amongst others. On screening there may be trapping of contrast during the stop test (Figures 4.20 and 6.2).

Treatment of bladder neck obstruction includes:

- Watchful waiting.
- α1-adrenoceptor antagonists:
  - Alfuzosin
  - Doxazosin
  - Tamsulosin
  - Terazosin.
- Trans-urethral incision of the bladder neck.

CLINICAL NOTE

The symptom of post-micturition dribble is usually not due to obstruction, but results from pooling of urine in the bulbar urethra and is common:

- if there is bladder neck obstruction
- in association with a urethral stricture or following urethroplasty
- with increasing age, presumably due to loss of elasticity of the urethra.

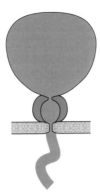

Figure 6.2 *Bladder neck obstruction/dyssynergia*, *showing trapping of contrast in the prostatic urethra during a stop test. During voiding the patient is instructed to stop his urinary stream: normally the contrast located in the prostatic urethra quickly milks back into the bladder; however, in patients with bladder neck dyssynergia, the tighter bladder neck resists retrograde flow, resulting in 'ballooning' of the prostatic urethra.*

Urethral stricture

Urethral strictures can occur in men of all ages and symptoms tend to only become evident when the urethral calibre is reduced to below 11 Fr. Strictures prevent the urethra from expanding and cause a characteristic constrictive picture on uroflowmetry (Figure 3.4e).

Causes of urethral stricture include:
- urethral trauma (injury, catheterization, surgery)
- urethral infection (usually sexually transmitted diseases)
- urethral inflammation
- urethral tumour (rare).

Although pressure/flow cystometry is useful in confirming BOO, more useful investigations include urethrography and cystoscopy which provide an anatomical assessment of the stricture (Figure 6.1e). Treatment is essentially surgical, usually with urethrotomy for simple short strictures or a urethroplasty for long, complex or recurrent strictures. Patients may require temporary bladder drainage via a catheter whilst awaiting surgery or if the surgery fails. Urethral dilatation is also helpful in keeping the urethra patent both prior to and following surgery.

Evaluation of suspected BOO

Initial evaluation of anatomical bladder outlet obstruction includes:
- **History:**
  - Character of symptoms (voiding versus storage)

133

○ Severity of symptoms:
  ▪ usually using a symptoms score such as IPSS or AUA-SI (Figure 6.3)
  ▪ impact on quality of life
○ Previous treatments
○ Current medications
○ Co-morbidities.
- **Examination:**
  ○ Abdomen for masses and palpable bladder
  ○ DRE for prostatic enlargement and signs of malignancy.
- **Investigations:**
  ○ Urine dipstix and or, MSU to rule out haematuria, pyuria or infection
  ○ PSA to screen for carcinoma and as a proxy for prostate size (only following appropriate counselling of the patient)
  ○ Uroflowmetry for characteristic pattern of poor voiding
  ○ PVR to assess for raised residuals or retention
  ○ Serum urea and electrolytes to assess renal function
  ○ Voiding diary to assess frequency and nocturia.

Further investigations should be performed if indicated including (but not limited to):
- pressure/flow cystometry
- abdominal/renal ultrasonography
- trans-rectal ultrasonography and prostatic biopsy
- cystoscopy
- urethrography.

Indications for urodynamics to assess BOO

Voiding diaries – Helpful in quantifying the symptoms of urgency, frequency and nocturia which are commonly associated with BOO and also occur in storage disorders such as OAB. May also be useful in ruling out suspected nocturnal polyuria particularly when the patient complains of significant nocturia (see Chapter 3).

Uroflowmetry and PVR – Can be used as a screening tool, and in most cases this is all that is required to confirm the presence of BOO (although it can't rule out a poorly contractile detrusor) before instigating treatment. In addition, it is a simple non-invasive test that can be used for subsequent

International Prostate Symptom Score (I-PSS)				(Please circle the appropriate score)		
	Not at all	Less than 1 time in 5	Less than half the time	About half the time	More than half the time	Almost always
1. Since the last visit, how often have you had a sensation of not emptying your bladder completely after you finished urinating?	0	1	2	3	4	5
2. Since the last visit, how often have you had to urinate again less than two hours after you finished urinating?	0	1	2	3	4	5
3. Since the last visit, how often have you found you stopped and started again several times when you urinated?	0	1	2	3	4	5
4. Since the last visit, how often have you found it difficult to postpone urination?	0	1	2	3	4	5
5. Since the last visit, how often have you had a weak urinary stream?	0	1	2	3	4	5
6. Since the last visit, how often have you had to push or strain to begin urination?	0	1	2	3	4	5
	None	1 time	2 times	3 times	4 times	5 or more times
7. Since the last visit, how many times did you most typically get up to urinate from the time you went to bed at night until the time you got up in the morning?	0	1	2	3	4	5
Total I-PS Score, S=						

Quality of life due to urinary symptoms				(Please circle the appropriate score)			
	Delighted	Pleased	Mostly satisfied	Mixed (about equally satisfied and dissatisfied)	Mostly dissatisfied	Unhappy	Terrible
1. If you were to spend the rest of your life with your urinary condition just the way it is now, how would you feel about that?	0	1	2	3	4	5	6
Quality of life assessment score =							

Figure 6.3 *International Prostate Symptom Score (IPSS).* This questionnaire is commonly used in the assessment of benign prostatic disease.

monitoring following therapy. Urethral strictures produce a characteristic pattern (Fig 3.4e), due to the constrictive obstruction, which may aid in making the diagnosis of stricture disease.

Pressure/flow cystometry – During voiding abnormally high pressures accompanied by a poor and prolonged urinary flow are characteristic of BOO. Cystometry is particularly useful in equivocal patients where it is necessary to rule out a detrusor cause for the LUTS, such as detrusor over-activity during the storage phase, or another cause for the dysfunctional voiding such as detrusor underactivity during the voiding phase. It is also important that any patient who is being considered for further surgery after initial failed surgery undergoes pressure/flow cystometry, both to confirm the symptoms are indeed due to BOO and to determine if any other complicating pathology is present such as DO.

Video urodynamics – This is the 'gold standard' investigation. Not only is all the information obtained as for pressure/flow cystometry but the added radiological screening allows the level of the obstruction to be determined. Enlargement of the prostate may be seen as a reduced calibre of the prostatic urethra and also as a prostatic indentation at the bladder base. Trapping of urine in the prostatic urethra due to bladder neck obstruction may also be visible during the stop test (Fig 6.2). Chronic changes to the bladder such as trabeculation and diverticula, as well as vesico-ureteric reflux during the high pressures generated by the bladder during voiding may also be seen (Table 6.1).

URODYNAMICS IN PRACTICE: PROSTATIC OBSTRUCTION

- Whilst there is a reasonable correlation between storage symptoms and DO, voiding symptoms correlate poorly with BOO.
- In most cases uroflowmetry and PVR estimation are sufficient to confirm a diagnosis of bladder outlet obstruction.
- Flow rate will not be able to differentiate between high detrusor pressure with low flow or low detrusor pressure with low flow – this distinction is important because many patients who have an unsatisfactory result following previous prostatic surgery have low pressure, low flow voiding dysfuction.
- Normal voiding may be maintained during the early stages of obstruction by a compensatory increase in voiding detrusor pressure.
- More detailed urodynamic investigation is essential if the flow rate is equivocal or if previous surgery has not led to any improvement or has left residual symptoms such as urgency or incontinence.

Urodynamic findings in BOO

Possible findings during urodynamic testing of patients with BOO

Voiding diaries	Increased daytime frequency Nocturia
Uroflowmetry and PVR	Initial hesitancy Prolonged flow time and voiding time Low Q_{max} (<15 ml/s) Low average flow rate Prolonged time to maximum flow Prolonged declining termination of flow Intermittent flow Raised PVR Characteristic low flow rate, long plateau in urethral stricture
Pressure/flow cystometry (Figures 6.4 and 6.5)	High opening pressure, Prolonged opening time High maximum detrusor pressure (often >60–100 cm H_2O) High pressure at maximum flow High closing pressure Low Q_{max} (<15 ml/s) Raised PVR Prolonged flow time Intermittent flow Abdominal straining to aid voiding Stop test – the isometric pressure contraction is often high (>50 cm H_2O), rarely able to perform due to the force of the detrusor contraction
Video urodynamics	Level of obstruction Calibre of urethra Stop test – trapping in prostatic urethra due to bladder neck obstruction Vesico-ureteric reflux Hydronephrosis Trabeculation Diverticula

Table 6.1 *Possible findings during urodynamic testing of patients with BOO*

Interpreting pressure/flow cystometry in BOO

It is usually obvious during the voiding phase of a pressure/flow urodynamic investigation that BOO is present. Many experts regard patients with a detrusor pressure >60 cm H_2O associated with a Q_{max} <10 mL/s to be urodynamically obstructed. The detrusor pressure often reaches

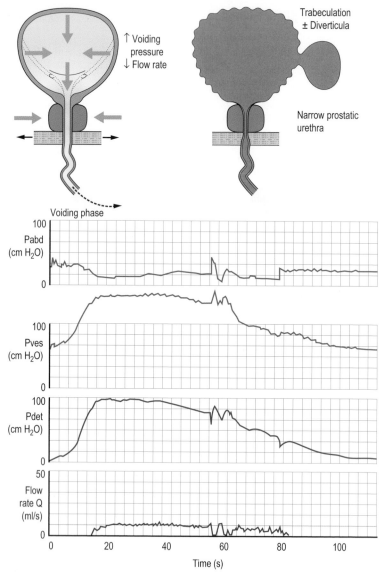

Figure 6.4 *Typical cystometry appearances for bladder outlet obstruction.* In this case the screening schematic shows obstruction at the level of the prostate.

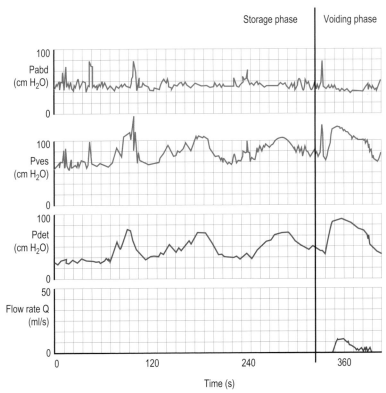

Figure 6.5 *Pressure/flow trace in patient with both detrusor overactivity during filling and BOO during voiding. This is a common pattern as many patients have both conditions coexisting.*

abnormally high levels (approaching or greater than 100 cm H_2O) in an attempt to expel the urine through the obstruction. Yet the flow rate remains low (often less than 8 ml/s) despite the elevated pressures (**high pressure, low flow**).

However in many cases the findings are more equivocal such as when:

- The elevated detrusor pressures ± abdominal straining are able to overcome the obstruction leading to a normal flow rate (**high pressure, normal flow**).
- The detrusor has not yet accommodated to the BOO and generates only normal pressures; or the detrusor muscle is failing (but has not yet become hypocontractile, acontractile) and is only able to generate pressures in the normal range but no higher. The result with both of these scenarios is poor flow (**normal/low pressure, low flow**).

139

To aid in determining if BOO is present the ICS pressure/flow nomogram can be used to calculate the bladder outlet obstruction index (BOOI) by plotting Q_{max} against $P_{det}@Q_{max}$. This will then categorize patients as being obstructed, unobstructed or equivocal. The ICS nomogram is based on a number of older nomograms (Abrams–Griffiths, Schafer LinPURR and URA nomograms) which were all found to have a high degree of correlation with each other; therefore only the ICS nomogram is required in routine clinical practice (Figure 6.6).

Modern urodynamic software usually contains the nomogram and will plot the data automatically; however if the nomogram is unavailable the BOOI (previously called the Abrams–Griffiths (AG) number) can be easily calculated manually using the following formula:

$$BOOI = P_{det}@Q_{max} - (2 \times Q_{max})$$

BOOI < 20 = unobstructed.
BOOI between 20 to 40 = equivocal.
BOOI > 40 = obstructed.

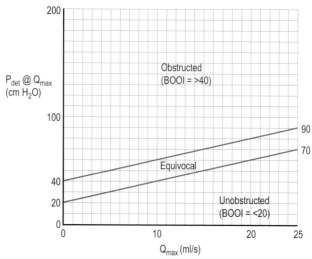

Figure 6.6 ICS BOO nomogram. Allows the BOOI to be easily calculated and the patient categorized as obstructed, unobstructed or equivocal. Must adjust for flow rate delay before using nomogram.

Example calculation:

If $P_{det}@Q_{max}$ is 100 cm H_2O and Q_{max} is 5 ml/s;

then the BOOI = $100 - (2 \times 5) = 90$ = obstructed

When using the nomogram and/or calculating the BOOI it must be remembered that the flow rate delay must be corrected for when calculating the $P_{det}@Q_{max}$, and this will depend on the local characteristics of the equipment (Chapter 4). It must also be borne in mind that the nomogram/BOOI was developed to assess male BOO due to a presumed prostatic cause. The nomogram and BOOI may therefore not be applicable in other situations such as in men with a functional obstruction (dyssynergia) and is not appropriate for women.

FUNCTIONAL OBSTRUCTION (DYSSYNERGIA)

During normal voiding the urethra relaxes synchronously with contraction of the detrusor muscle. Should the urethra and in particular its associated sphincter mechanisms fail to relax during voiding then uncoordinated activity between the detrusor and the urethra/sphincter occurs; this is termed dyssynergia. The ICS has defined a number of patterns of functional obstruction:

Dysfunctional voiding – 'An intermittent and/or fluctuating flow rate due to involuntary intermittent contractions of the peri-urethral striated muscle during voiding, in neurologically normal patients'. The condition occurs most frequently in children and it is thought to be due to intermittent pelvic floor contractions. (The old term for this was 'non-neurogenic, neurogenic bladder'.) Poor relaxation of the pelvic floor and urethral sphincter mechanism is also common in patients with voiding dysfunction, especially those with pelvic pain syndrome.

Detrusor sphincter dyssnergia (DSD) – 'A detrusor contraction concurrent with an involuntary contraction of the urethral and/or peri-urethral striated muscle' (Figure 6.1c). The condition tends to occur in patients with a supra-sacral neurological lesion, for example a spinal cord injury, Parkinson's disease and also multiple sclerosis (MS) (see Chapter 9). Co-existing DSD and prostatic obstruction can occur in elderly men such as those with Parkinson's disease and can be particularly difficult to manage. A useful therapeutic manoeuvre in such a situation can be to insert a temporary intra-urethral prostatic stent to treat the prostate obstruction, thus allowing the two conditions to be differentiated.

Non-relaxing urethral sphincter obstruction – 'A non-relaxing, obstructing urethra resulting in reduced urine flow' tends to occur in patients with a sacral or infra-sacral neurological lesion, i.e. meningomyelocoele or following radical pelvic surgery which has damaged the innervation.

Fowler's syndrome – This is an uncommon condition that primarily affects young women in their 20–30s, in whom the urethral sphincter mechanism fails to relax leading to raised PVRs and retention. There may be a history of lifelong voiding difficulty and often there is associated secondary detrusor failure. Many of these women have an associated hormonal problem (Stein–Leventhal syndrome – hirsutism, polycystic ovary syndrome and amenorrhoea). The aetiology is unknown and the gold standard investigation for this condition is a sphincter electromyogram (EMG), although pressure/flow cystometry, urethral pressure profilometry and ultrasound sphincter volume measurement may also be valuable. Some women may spontaneously recover whilst in others it may be a lifelong condition. CISC may be required to ensure adequate bladder drainage although it is poorly correlated and sacral neuromodulation has also been found to be of some benefit in restoring voiding.

Evaluation of suspected functional obstruction

The brief descriptions given above should be borne in mind when evaluating any patient who has outflow obstruction. Associated neurological symptoms and signs should suggest the possibility of DSD or a non-relaxing urethral sphincter obstruction.

These conditions are best evaluated using video urodynamics with synchronous use of electromyography and should ideally be performed in units with specialist expertise in investigating and managing these conditions.

Urodynamic findings in functional obstruction

Urodynamic findings are similar to those seen in anatomical BOO and are characterized by high detrusor pressures coupled with poor flow. With DSD the sphincter may intermittently open and close during voiding. When the sphincter is open the detrusor pressures may be normal or moderately high. If the sphincter suddenly closes during a void the detrusor pressure rises because the detrusor is now iso-volumetrically contracting against the closed sphincter (similar to a stop test); the flow rate will also reduce/stop whilst the sphincter is closed. When the

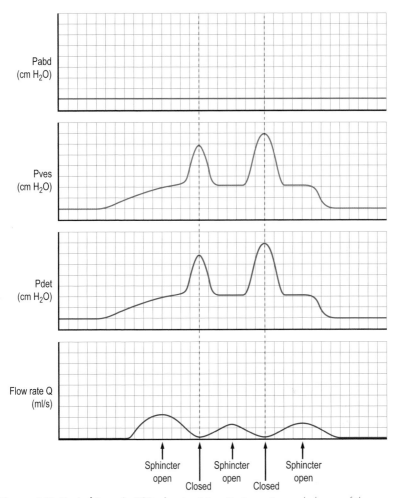

Figure 6.7 *Typical trace in DSD,* showing intermittent opening and closure of the urethral sphincter causing a characteristic flow pattern and pressure changes.

sphincter re-opens the detrusor pressures will drop and the flow will be re-established. This pattern may be repeated a number of times during a void (Figure 6.7).

Video urodynamics will also show the intermittent sphincter activity and the level of the obstruction. In addition the bladder may develop chronic changes due to the elevated voiding pressures including trabeculation, diverticula and vesico-ureteric reflux (most noticeable when the sphincter closes, causing a significant rise in detrusor pressure). The bladder and urethra in females may develop a 'spinning top'

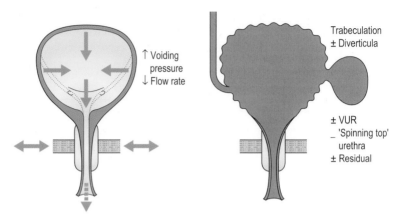

Figure 6.8 *Video appearances in DSD.* High pressure and low flow from sphincter obstruction may lead to chronic changes. VUR, vesico-ureteric reflux.

appearance due to widening of the posterior urethra due to the chronic high pressure trapping of urine in the urethra above the sphincter when the sphincter closes (Figure 6.8). EMG studies concurrent with pressure/flow cystometry may also show intermittent sphincteric activity during voiding.

DETRUSOR FAILURE (UNDERACTIVE DETRUSOR FUNCTION)

In addition to anatomical or functional obstruction to urine outflow, detrusor failure can also cause voiding dysfunction in both men and women.

Poor detrusor function during voiding can be classified as:

- **Detrusor underactivity** – Where the contraction of the detrusor is of reduced strength and/or duration, resulting in prolonged bladder emptying and/or failure to achieve complete bladder emptying within a normal time span. This was previously termed as a 'hypo-contractile' detrusor.
- **Acontractile detrusor** – where the detrusor cannot be demonstrated to contract during urodynamic assessment.

Causes of detrusor failure include:

- **Primary:**
  - idiopathic.
- **Secondary:**
  - neurogenic bladder dysfunction (usually lower motor neuron)
  - bladder outlet obstruction.

Frequently patients present with chronic retention ± overflow incontinence, but detrusor failure should be considered in all patients who present with voiding difficulty. A uroflowmetry and PVR estimation is a good screening tool for the condition. An intermittent straining pattern or sometimes a prolonged, low flow rate void associated with a raised PVR should raise suspicions of detrusor failure (although a similar picture is frequently seen with BOO). However, only pressure/flow cystometry can definitively differentiate between BOO and detrusor failure and should therefore be performed in all equivocal cases, especially if the PVR is abnormally raised.

Chronic retention – This is a non-painful distended bladder, which remains palpable or percussable after the patient has passed urine.

Elderly men in particular are at risk of developing chronic retention secondary to BOO, but any of the causes of detrusor failure may lead to chronic retention. Often the cause of the chronic retention is unknown (idiopathic). A small group of middle-aged to elderly women present with acute retention of urine, usually after surgery and commonly vigorously deny any previous history of voiding difficulty. In addition, some women report 'chronic holding' either due to busy schedules or in an attempt to avoid public restrooms. Urodynamic investigation sometimes demonstrates an underactive detrusor with chronic retention in this distinct group.

Management of detrusor failure

Initial – The initial management of underactive detrusor is aimed at ensuring that the bladder is adequately drained, thus preventing overdistension of the bladder and overstretching of the detrusor muscle fibres leading to further damage; and also preventing the development or worsening of damage to the upper urinary tracts.

Bladder drainage can be achieved by:
- Clean intermittent self-catheterization (CISC) – preferred option.
- Indwelling catheterization:
  ○ Urethral
  ○ Supra-pubic (preferable to long-term urethral catheterization) – particularly useful in patients with a suspected reversible neurological disorder, as it allows the serial assessment of PVRs to assess ability to void spontaneously.

Long term – The long term management of detrusor underactivity is directed at the correction of any underlying aetiology, if possible. If the underlying cause is adequately treated and the bladder is allowed a period of 'rest' with suitable drainage then there may be some recovery of detrusor function. Bladder training can also be useful, particularly for the 'infrequent voiders' who are instructed to void by the clock (e.g. 2-hourly).

In a man with detrusor failure secondary to prostatic BOO a period of drainage may allow detectable function to return; in such a situation proceeding to prostatic surgery may be appropriate, whereas if there is no improvement in detrusor function then the voiding symptoms are unlikely to resolve and the man is likely to continue to need the bladder draining artificially following prostatic surgery.

Urodynamics in detrusor failure

Uroflowmetry and PVR – A useful screening and monitoring tool. A prolonged flow is usually seen along with a low Q_{max}. Often the flow is intermittent and the patient may be attempting to void with abdominal straining. The PVR will be consistently raised (usually above 200–300 ml). The flow rate pattern is similar to the pattern seen in BOO and it is impossible to be sure if voiding dysfunction is due to detrusor failure or BOO on the basis of this test. Though an elevated PVR suggests decompensation and relative underactivity of the detrusor, and not BOO.

Pressure/flow cystometry – This is able to determine if detrusor underactivity is present. During the storage phase the bladder may be hypo-sensitive with late bladder sensations detected and a high cystometric capacity. The patient may not demonstrate a strong desire to void and so may not have a measurable maximum cystometric capacity. In such cases the cystometric capacity (at which filling is stopped) may need to be determined by the investigator. On being given permission to void the patient often has a long delay before initiating the void. The detrusor pressure only rises minimally (or not at all if acontractile) with a corresponding low flow rate (**low pressure, low flow voiding**). Often the patient has to perform abdominal straining to initiate or maintain a void. Frequently only a negligible amount of fluid is voided (Figure 6.9).

Video urodynamics – This is useful to determine if there is any reflux of contrast at any point during the study and may also show hydronephrosis if there is any upper tract damage. Video urodynamics is therefore particularly important in patients with suspected neurogenic dysfunction. If sufficient contrast is voided then it may be possible to see the level of obstruction if the detrusor failure is secondary to BOO; although in many cases this is not possible due to the negligible volume voided.

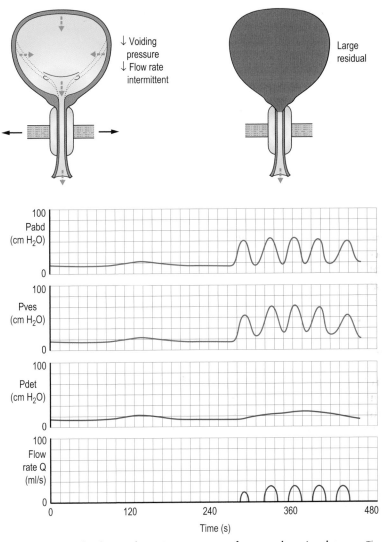

Figure 6.9 *Typical video urodynamic appearances for an underactive detrusor.* The trace shows virtually no detrusor activity. The patient has voided small amounts by intermittent abdominal straining.

URODYNAMICS IN PRACTICE: DETRUSOR FAILURE AND OUTLET RESISTANCE

It must be remembered that a *normal* detrusor contraction will be recorded as:

- high pressure if the outlet is obstructed
- normal pressure if there is normal outlet resistance
- low pressure if there is low outlet resistance.

Therefore patients with apparent detrusor underactivity may have a very low outlet resistance, as may occur if the sphincteric mechanisms are grossly incompetent.

A patient with a very low outlet resistance is likely to experience stress incontinence during the filling phase.

CHAPTER 7

Sensory disorders

INTRODUCTION

Urodynamic investigations were originally developed to study the 'motor' function of the lower urinary tract. However in recent years it has been recognized that the sensory component of voiding function is frequently involved in the pathophysiology of common lower urinary tract disorders such as the overactive bladder (OAB) syndrome. Bladder sensation can be assessed using stimulating electrodes introduced through the urethra, but such techniques are used for research purposes rather than routine assessment.

Urodynamic investigations are not ideal techniques for evaluating sensory disorders, which can be very subjective, but do allow some sensory information to be obtained and enable the observer to:

- measure the sensory thresholds objectively
- exclude motor disorders.

Abnormalities of bladder sensation can be broadly categorized into:

- increased bladder sensation (hyper-sensitive)
- reduced bladder sensation (hypo-sensitive).

HYPER-SENSITIVITY

Increased bladder sensation – This is defined, during filling cystometry, as an early first sensation of bladder filling (or an early desire to void) and/or an early strong desire to void, which occurs at low bladder volume and which persists.

Causes of hyper-sensitivity include:

- Idiopathic.
- Bladder or urethral inflammation:
  - bacterial cystitis
  - urethritis
  - urethral syndrome
  - post-irradiation cystitis
  - cyclophosphamide cystitis
  - chemical cystitis.

- Chronic prostatitis.
- Bladder pain syndrome/painful bladder syndrome/interstitial cystitis (BPS/PBS/IC).
- Bladder calculus.
- Bladder carcinoma.

Bacterial cystitis is the commonest cause; it is therefore important to ensure that there is no concurrent infection immediately before performing pressure/flow urodynamics, as the test will often exacerbate the urinary infection and will produce a falsely increased bladder sensitivity.

Evaluation of bladder hyper-sensitivity

Frequently patients with bladder hyper-sensitivity complain of storage symptoms and also supra-pubic pain in association with bladder filling.

A full history is particularly important in the assessment of hyper-sensitive disorders of the bladder. Clinical features can include:

- **Daytime frequency** – a prominent symptom for which bladder pain rather than impending incontinence is the trigger.
- **Urgency** – but rarely associated with incontinence.
- **Bladder pain** – usually relieved by voiding.
- **Dysuria.**
- **Dyspareunia** – a common symptom.
- **Haematuria** – requires full investigation of both the lower and upper urinary tracts.

The symptoms are usually chronic, often with a history of previous probable urinary tract infections; although frequently urine cultures have not been performed or the urine has been found to be sterile. Antibiotics have usually been unhelpful in providing long term relief from the symptoms. Women often report improvement at the end of their menstrual cycle and many will have had a hysterectomy, perhaps for lower abdominal/pelvic pain, but with no obvious gynaecological pathology.

Examination may be unremarkable, but attention should be paid to the urethral meatus, which may be inflamed or show mucosal prolapse (a urethral caruncle). There may also be bladder tenderness, both suprapubically and on vaginal examination. A gentle bimanual examination will identify other pelvic pathology. The iliococcygeus muscle or pelvic side wall is often tender and trigger points may be identified.

All cases require urinalysis and culture to rule out an active UTI or haematuria. Often other investigations are indicated to exclude other causes for the symptoms including:

- urine cytology
- voiding diaries
- pressure/flow cystometry
- cystoscopy ± biopsy
- abdominal/pelvic ultrasound (to rule out gynaecological disorders).

Investigations of bladder oversensitivity are often complex with the requirement to exclude a number of pathologies. Figure 7.1 shows a possible management pathway for the investigation and management of this complex problem.

Management is also often difficult and options for bladder hypersensitivity and suspected BPS/PBS/IC include:

- Cystoscopy and overdistension (pressure of 80–100 cm H_2O for 5 min) and bladder biopsies of any abnormality as appropriate – this procedure is both investigative and in some cases therapeutic. There is usually a rise in pulse rate and blood pressure in patients with bladder hyper-sensitivity, under a light general anaesthetic; in addition, bleeding and non-specific glomerulations can often be seen in the bladder following the distension.
- Urethral recalibration up to 42 Fr – may improve symptoms if there is an associated urethral hyper-sensitivity.
- Intra-vesical installations may be helpful in some patients:
  - dimethyl sulphoxide (DMSO)
  - heparinoid agents (either alone or in combination with lidocaine and bicarbonate)
  - steroids
  - hyaluronic acid.
- Self-help groups (local and national).
- Diet and fluid intake manipulation.
- Medications:
  - non-steroidal anti-inflammatories
  - analgesics
  - anticholinergics
  - antidepressants
  - antihistamines
  - H_2 antagonists
  - pentosan polysulphate sodium
  - corticosteroids.
- Surgery (if symptoms are intractable and debilitating):
  - cystectomy
  - entero-cystoplasty.

It must be remembered that the evidence base for the clinical effectiveness of any of these therapies is very limited. Treatment of bladder hyper-

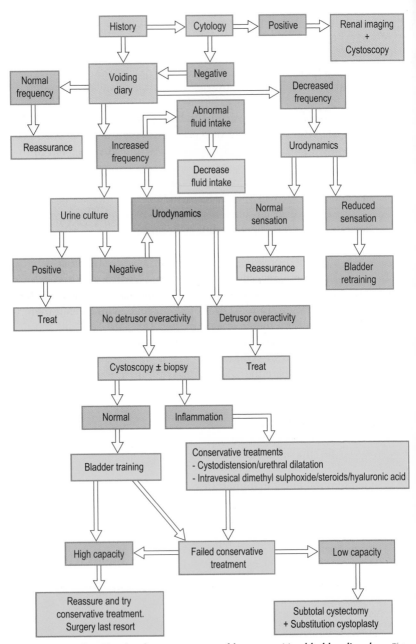

Figure 7.1 Algorithm for the management of hyper-sensitive bladder disorders. *This is a complex area and such an algorithm usually has to be modified for each individual patient.*

sensitivity due to infection or mucosal inflammation is beyond the scope of this book.

Urodynamics in bladder hyper-sensitivity

The diagnosis of a hyper-sensitive bladder is one of exclusion, relying particularly upon the exclusion of intra-vesical pathology in particular overt malignancy or carcinoma in situ.

Voiding diaries – Are useful in this condition for determining the daytime frequency, which is often significantly raised, typically frequency is raised more than in patients with overactive bladder. However the results often vary considerably from week to week and it is essential not to base therapy on the results of voiding diaries alone.

Pressure/flow cystometry – Is particularly useful both in excluding other causes for the symptoms including detrusor overactivity (DO) and also in diagnosing increased bladder sensation. Premature bladder sensations usually occur in quick succession culminating in bladder discomfort and the strong desire to void, thereby reducing the capacity. In addition, patients with hyper-sensitive painful bladders often demonstrate high urethral closure pressures at rest and during voiding, increased EMG activity with voiding, and high voiding pressures.

URODYNAMICS IN PRACTICE: HYPER-SENSITIVE BLADDER

- All patients who have symptoms suggestive of a hyper-sensitive bladder should have urine culture and if negative an urodynamic assessment.
- Urodynamics is helpful in diagnosing patients who have hyper-sensitive painful bladders and also helps exclude other conditions such as detrusor overactivity.
- Catheterization may be painful – passage of the catheter through the urethra and contact with the bladder mucosa may cause pain suggesting the urethral syndrome.
- Major diagnostic features are premature first sensation of filling, premature first and strong desire to void. There is a reduced maximum cystometric capacity (MCC) due to bladder discomfort.
- High voiding pressure associated with increased EMG activity.
- High urethral pressure at rest and during voiding.
- Filling pressures and voiding function may be normal.
- The diagnosis of a 'hyper-sensitive bladder' is one of exclusion and relies upon the exclusion of other intra-vesical pathology including malignancy.

HYPO-SENSITIVE BLADDER

Reduced bladder sensation – This is defined, during filling cystometry, as diminished sensation throughout bladder filling.

Causes of hypo-sensitivity include:

- **Idiopathic.**
- **Neurogenic:**
  - spinal cord injury (SCI)
  - pelvic trauma
  - radical hysterectomy
  - abdomino-perineal (AP) resection of the rectum
  - peripheral neuropathy (e.g. diabetes).
- **Secondary:**
  - chronic retention (see Chapter 6).

Due to the loss of desire to micturate, patients with a hypo-sensitive bladder often retain large volumes within the bladder and only infrequently void. This leads to chronic overdistension and eventually the development of detrusor failure. Conversely detrusor failure due to other causes can also lead to painless chronic retention with resultant reduced bladder sensitivity. Therefore bladder hypo-sensitivity and detrusor failure frequently co-exist and are intimately related (see Chapter 6).

Neurogenic hypo-sensitivity is usually due to denervation of the sensory pathways such as occurs with spinal cord injury or with local disruption to the nerves during pelvic surgery. Idiopathic hypo-sensitivity predominantly affects female patients with no other lower urinary tract pathology (and who commonly report 'holding' urination) and this condition is sometimes referred to as 'camel bladder'.

Evaluation of bladder hypo-sensitivity

Often patients who have a hypo-sensitive bladder have no other symptoms apart from the loss of the desire to micturate. Other symptoms can include:

- straining to urinate with a poor flow
- a feeling of incomplete emptying
- infrequent voiding
- urinary frequency and incontinence secondary to poor bladder emptying
- recurrent urinary tract infections
- history of chronic retention.

There may also be a history of neurological injury (spinal cord or cauda equina), pelvic surgery or diabetes. Most patients with neurological trauma usually have associated detrusor failure.

Examination may reveal impaired sensation on testing the sacral dermatomes and also raised PVRs.

Management of bladder hypo-sensitivity

It is important that the bladder is adequately drained to prevent the progression to detrusor failure or upper tract damage. Treatment choices are:

- **Bladder training** – If the patient is able to void spontaneously then they should be encouraged to void 'by the clock' about six times a day and double void even though the desire to void may be absent. If such treatment is started early in the course of the condition it may prevent subsequent impairment of detrusor function. It is important to monitor these patients carefully to check that they do not develop silent 'chronic retention' with increasing PVRs.

- **Alpha-adrenergic antagonists** – The success of alpha-adrenergic antagonists in improving the efficiency of voiding is limited, but empirical therapy may be of benefit.

- **Clean intermittent self-catheterization (CISC)** – If the patient is unable to initiate voiding or if voiding is inefficient with raised PVRs then CISC should be performed.

Urodynamics in bladder hypo-sensitivity

Voiding diaries – Are useful in identifying infrequent voiding and the patient's functional bladder capacity may be significantly increased. Diaries may also be therapeutic when used in conjunction with bladder training.

Uroflowmetry and PVR – Not usually useful to investigate altered the sensation but if there is any detrusor failure then there may be poor voiding with a straining pattern and raised PVRs.

Pressure/flow cystometry – Diagnosis of hypo-sensitivity is dependent on increased volumes at which sensations occur; usually there is also a high cystometric capacity. There may be no strong desire to void and often the urodynamicist will have to decide when to stop filling. In many cases there are no sensations felt throughout filling. If only hypo-sensitivity is present then the voiding phase should be normal; however, if there is any associated detrusor failure then voiding may be prolonged, intermittent and inefficient with no or minimal increase in detrusor pressure; a low pressure, low flow pattern (see Chapter 6).

URODYNAMICS IN PRACTICE: HYPO-SENSITIVE BLADDER

- The characteristic urodynamic features are an increase in the volume at which the first sensation, first desire and strong desire to void occur, often with an associated high cystometric capacity.
- In severe cases there may be almost no bladder sensation and voiding needs to be initiated without any desire to micturate 'by the clock'.
- In pure hypo-sensitivity, detrusor function during filling and voiding is normal.
- Detrusor failure may be a cause or consequence of bladder hypo-sensitivity and results in the inability to generate a detrusor contraction and often results in a high PVR.

CHAPTER 8

The contracted bladder

INTRODUCTION

Bladder contracture is the end stage of chronic inflammatory disorders of the bladder or results from the treatment of carcinoma such as post radiotherapy. The chronic fibrotic damage to the bladder causes the bladder function to deteriorate severely.

Causes of fibrotic contracture include:
- prior bladder carcinoma treated by multiple resections
- surgery
- radiation therapy
- tuberculosis
- chemical cystitis
- severe sensory bladder disorders
- schistosomiasis.

Often fibrotic contracture is preceded by inflammation so bladder hypersensitivity and contracture may co-exist. However, the final stage of the condition may not be associated with hyper-sensitivity.

HISTORY AND EXAMINATION

The patient will usually have a previous long history of treatment for bladder carcinoma or chronic bladder inflammation. Symptoms of contracture can include:
- **Daytime frequency and nocturia** – usually the predominant complaint.
- **Urgency** – often present.
- **Stress incontinence** – often present.
- **Bladder pain** – during filling if there is active inflammation of the bladder.

Examination is usually unremarkable although there may be some supra-pubic tenderness.

MANAGEMENT

In most cases, treatment of the underlying cause will have already failed to halt disease progression and therefore operative treatment is indicated. Most cases of contracture are treated by cystectomy and urinary diversion or bladder reconstruction (see Chapter 5). More conservative treatments such as cysto-distension do not produce long term symptomatic relief.

Urodynamics in bladder contracture

Pressure/flow cystometry – Bladder contracture is best assessed with video urodynamics. Often during the filling phase there is a reduction in the volumes at which bladder sensations such as the first sensation of filling occur and the maximum cystometric capacity (MCC) is also reduced, giving the urodynamic appearance of bladder hyper-sensitivity. The compliance of the bladder is also often severely reduced, due to fibrosis of the detrusor muscle (Chapter 4). The findings must be interpreted in the context of data from a bladder diary and an assessment of anatomical bladder capacity.

In some instances there may be fibrosis around the bladder neck, thereby preventing adequate closure during filling and leading to incontinence. The incontinence may be due to the pressure rise in the bladder secondary to poor compliance or may be due to increased transmission of intra-abdominal pressure (stress incontinence). In patients considering an entero-cystoplasty, the outlet should be urodynamically assessed for the presence of intrinsic sphincter deficiency and the subsequent need for surgical correction at the time of bladder augmentation. Frequently there is fibrosis around the ureteric orifices, preventing closure with resultant vesico-ureteric reflux. In severe cases the upper tracts may act as a 'reservoir' for urine (with gross hydronephrosis) and may hold far more urine than the bladder.

Voiding may also be affected; fibrosis of the detrusor will lead to inefficient contractions and detrusor underactivity (Chapter 6). The result will be a weak detrusor contraction coupled with a poor flow rate, prolonged voiding and raised PVR; often the patient uses abdominal straining to aid voiding (low pressure, low flow voiding).

Video screening will not only determine if incontinence or vesico-ureteric reflux is present but usually shows that the bladder is small and unusually spherical in appearance (Figure 8.1).

URODYNAMICS IN PRACTICE: THE CONTRACTED BLADDER

Frequent urodynamic findings include:
- Reduction in first sensation volume.
- Reduction in first desire and strong desire volume.
- Reduced cystometric capacity.
- Reduced bladder compliance.
- Incontinence.
- Vesico-ureteric reflux and hydronephrosis.
- Detrusor underactivity with inefficient voiding (low pressure, low flow voiding).
- Raised PVR.
- Compensatory abdominal straining during voiding.
- Small, 'spherical' bladder on screening.

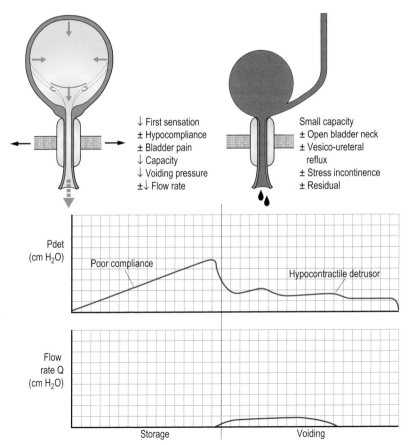

Figure 8.1 *Typical urodynamic appearances for a contracted bladder,* summarizing the varied features that may be present on video urodynamics.

Urodynamics following cystoplasty

Entero-cystoplasty is a major operative treatment for bladder dysfunction such as intractable detrusor overactivity, painful bladder syndrome/ interstitial cystitis, post-irradiation fibrosis and tuberculosis. During this procedure the bladder is opened as in clam cystoplasty and a small or large bowel segment is opened (detubularized) and patched onto the bladder. This serves to increase the bladder capacity.

All patients for whom such a procedure is planned should undergo careful urodynamic evaluation before the operation; to establish a baseline for detrusor and bladder outlet function, to predict post-procedure complications and exclude any other causes for the LUTS.

Following cystoplasty bowel peristalsis in the segment patched to the bladder frequently occurs and voiding is usually accomplished by abdominal straining, which is more efficient when co-ordinated with the peristaltic contractions. Unfortunately, some patients experience persistent or new symptoms such as urgency, daytime frequency, incontinence, voiding difficulty or recurrent UTIs. Video urodynamics is important in the evaluation of post-cystoplasty problems and attention should be paid to several important factors:

- Is the cystoplasty overactive?
- Is this overactivity associated with outflow obstruction?
- Is incontinence due to hyperactivity of the bowel segment or impaired outflow resistance?
- PVR should also be measured, usually by ultrasound bladder scanning.
- Are the continuing symptoms due to persistence of the underlying sensory bladder problem, where cystectomy and another form of cystoplasty or diversion may be appropriate?

Management

Overactive cystoplasties associated with outflow obstruction are best treated by first relieving the obstruction:

- in females this usually means urethral dilatation
- in males bladder neck incision or trans-urethral prostatectomy (TURP) may be indicated.

Overactive cystoplasties without obstruction are best treated by pharmacotherapy initially. Anticholinergic therapy is usually used, as are antispasmodic drugs such as mebeverine, although drug therapy may not be successful. If drug therapy fails a further detubularization procedure to add a patch of small bowel to the side of the cystoplasty may be helpful; this reduces the activity of the cystoplasty and allows many patients, particularly females, to void to completion by abdominal straining and thereby minimising adverse symptoms. However, underactive cystoplasties can be associated with a large PVR, which in turn can lead to recurrent UTIs. This problem is more likely to occur in males, in whom outflow resistance is higher and where abdominal straining is less efficient; in such cases CISC may be required.

CHAPTER 9

Neurogenic bladder disorders

INTRODUCTION

Neurogenic bladder dysfunction describes abnormal function of the bladder and urethra due to lesions affecting their innervation, either within the central nervous system or in the peripheral nerves of the lower urinary tract.

Neurological conditions can alter bladder and urethral function by altering:

- detrusor activity
- striated muscle sphincter activity
- smooth muscle sphincter activity
- bladder and urethral sensation.

PATTERNS OF NEUROGENIC DYSFUNCTION

Although each individual patient will have a unique pattern of lower urinary tract dysfunction and require an individual management plan, the site of the lesion gives an indication of the likely pattern of the dysfunction.

Neurological lesions can be divided into four broad anatomical areas:

1. Suprapontine.
2. Pontine (brainstem).
3. Suprasacral spinal cord.
4. Sacral-subsacral (peripheral nerve and cauda equina).

Suprapontine

Causes – Typically suprapontine disorders are due to cerebro-vascular accidents (CVA), brain tumours, head injury, dementia and cerebral palsy.

Pattern of dysfunction – Neurogenic detrusor overactivity (NDO) commonly occurs due to reduced cortical inhibitory control of the micturition reflex. As the pontine co-ordination centres are unaffected by this lesion, detrusor and sphincter function co-ordination is preserved; for this reason, patients with suprapontine lesions usually do not develop high pressure neurogenic bladders. However many patients appropriately increase sphincter activity during DO to avoid urgency incontinence, and this increase in EMG activity has been coined pseudodyssynergia. In addition, some patients with cortical lesions lose the ability to voluntarily void and others lose the sensation of bladder fullness and urgency.

Pontine

Causes – Typically pontine disorders are due to Parkinson's disease, multiple system atrophy (MSA) and multiple sclerosis (MS).

Pattern of dysfunction – The brainstem contains both the pontine micturition centre (PMC) and the pontine storage centre (PSC); therefore a lesion in this area can cause of variety of storage and voiding dysfunctions to occur simultaneously. These include NDO, detrusor underactivity, detrusor sphincter dyssynergia (DSD) and external sphincter relaxation.

Suprasacral spinal cord

Causes – Typically suprasacral spinal cord disorders are due to spinal cord injury (SCI) and MS.

Pattern of dysfunction – Due to the loss of higher detrusor inhibition and co-ordination of voiding these patients typically have DO associated with DSD. Bladder filling sensation will also be lost in a complete SCI. Spontaneous reflex voiding can occur; however it is uncontrolled and associated with incontinence. DSD may lead to high voiding pressure and upper tract damage and this is a particularly 'dangerous' pattern of urological dysfunction; it is classically seen in high level (cervical cord) lesions.

Sacral and subsacral

Causes – Typically from myelomeningocoele, spina bifida, MS, diabetes mellitus and iatrogenic from surgical injury.

Pattern of dysfunction – A variety of patterns of dysfunction are seen depending on the level of the lesion and the extent of the denervation. A complete sacral or subsacral lesion will lead to an acontractile detrusor, incompetent urethra and loss of bladder sensation. A complete lesion around the conus may demonstrate an acontractile detrusor with a normal or overactive urethra. A complete lumbo-sacral lesion may cause an overactive detrusor with an incompetent urethra. Most lesions are however incomplete and depending on the pathways disrupted can give a varying pattern of dysfunction, e.g. injury to the pudendal nerves may lead to an incompetent urethra whereas an injury to the pelvic nerves may lead to an underactive detrusor with impaired bladder sensation but with a normally functioning urethra. Injury to the afferent axons and pathways may lead to diminished bladder sensation. In addition, incomplete lesions can result in neurogenic detrusor overactivity and high pressure neurogenic bladders.

URODYNAMICS FOR NEUROGENIC BLADDER DISORDERS

In the management of neurogenic lower urinary tract function:
- The primary aim is to protect the upper urinary tract:
  ○ to maintain low intra-vesical pressures
  ○ to maintain a low post-void residual.
- The secondary aims are to improve the quality of life and/or achieve continence.

Urodynamic investigations can characterize the nature of the detrusor and sphincteric abnormality to:
- identify those patients who are at risk of upper tract damage
- formulate the best treatment strategies to achieve efficient bladder emptying and continence and reduce the incidence of urinary tract infections and autonomic dysreflexia.

Many patients with neurological disorders don't display symptoms or signs until significant damage has occurred to the upper tracts or to detrusor function. Frequently urodynamic findings in this group of patients do not correlate well with the neurological examination findings and therefore the examination findings should not be used to plan the urological management. Instead all patients with neurological dysfunction that affects or is likely to affect lower urinary tract function should receive a thorough urodynamic assessment at an early stage to fully characterize the function and to plan appropriate management; patients may require subsequent follow-up urodynamic investigations to determine the success of any intervention and the extent of any change in lower urinary tract function.

Assessment of lower urinary tract dysfunction is no different from that in neurologically normal patients, consisting of history, examination, voiding diaries, uroflowmetry and pressure flow studies (±EMG). However the interpretation is often more complex and there are specific hazards such as autonomic dysreflexia; therefore the investigations are best performed in specialist centres using video urodynamics. It must be remembered that patients with neurogenic bladder dysfunction also suffer from the same lower urinary tract disorders as the rest of the population, e.g. BOO related to the prostate, and these conditions may further complicate assessment and management. Management should be tailored for each patient depending on the pattern of dysfunction and a plan for follow-up, other relevant investigations (renal function, ultrasound) and repeat urodynamic assessments should be carried out.

NDO AND SPHINCTER OVERACTIVITY (DSD)

The presence of both NDO and sphincter overactivity is a particularly dangerous urodynamic situation and as a rule of thumb those patients with a competent bladder outflow and a pre-micturition pressure of 40 cm H_2O or higher are at particular risk of developing upper urinary tract problems due to the high backpressure, although this is by no means an absolute value and damage to the upper tracts can occur at lower pressures (Figure 9.1). If this pattern of dysfunction is present then the preservation of renal function is of the utmost importance; this requires control of both the NDO and the sphincter overactivity.

Treatment strategies for the NDO include:

- anticholinergics
- botulinum toxin therapy to the bladder

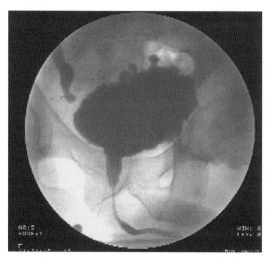

Figure 9.1 *Video urodynamic screening in a spinal cord injured patient,* showing obstruction at the level of the sphincter (DSD), right vesico-ureteric reflux and hydronephrosis and also multiple bladder diverticuli.

- neuromodulation
- bladder surgery such as augmentation.

Treatment strategies for the overactive sphincter are to ensure adequate drainage; these include:
- clean intermittent self-catheterization (CISC)
- botulinum toxin therapy to the sphincter
- neuromodulation
- intra-urethral stents
- sphincterotomy.

Incontinence that occurs as a result of a sphincterotomy or stent insertion can be controlled by implanting an artificial urinary sphincter.

The patient should at the least have annual urodynamic assessments, PVRs and kidney function tests performed and the patient should be followed up according to recognized guidelines such as those produced by the International Consultation on Incontinence (ICI).

SPINAL SHOCK

Patients who have lesions above the sacral micturition centre initially go through a period of spinal shock in which there is loss of neurological (reflex) activity below the level of the injury. This usually results in complete urinary retention due to an acontractile detrusor and also to the maintenance of some residual sphincteric competence. Until there is recovery of some neurological activity the patient will require either indwelling or intermittent catheterization.

URODYNAMICS IN PRACTICE: NEUROGENIC BLADDER DYSFUNCTION

- Initial urodynamic studies are most commonly performed after the spinal shock period is over (usually 3–4 months after spinal cord injury) when reflex activity is re-established, along with a baseline renal ultrasound or intravenous urography.
- Routine urodynamics and renal radiography are usually performed annually or every alternate year depending upon the nature of the vesico-urethral dysfunction.
- Indications for non-routine urodynamic investigation in patients with neurogenic disorders include symptomatic voiding dysfunction, urinary incontinence, renal deterioration (renal scarring, hydronephrosis, elevated serum creatinine),

recurrent urinary tract infections, a change in voiding pattern and the onset of autonomic dysreflexia.

Technique

- Many authorities recommend not emptying the bladder before commencing filling cystometry in patients who have NDO because these patients usually have persistently high PVRs and rapid bladder evacuation may alter the characteristics of the detrusor overactivity and result in an over-diagnosis of poor bladder compliance.
- Residual urine estimation by catheter or ultrasound should be obtained at another time when emptying is more physiological.
- Some patients improve emptying during urodynamics by abdominal straining, supra-pubic compression or triggering reflex detrusor contractions by perineal or abdominal tapping.
- The filling rate should be slow, so as to not provoke premature detrusor overactivity which may potentially mask information regarding sensations, cystometric capacity and compliance. Rapid filling may also trigger DSD as well as over-diagnose poor bladder compliance. In addition, 30 seconds at the end of filling should be allowed for bladder accommodation before interpreting the pre-micturition pressure.
- Observation of several filling–voiding cycles is recommended to accurately define bladder and urethral abnormalities – the first voiding sequence may be altered by passing the catheter, which may precipitate or inhibit detrusor overactivity and be unrepresentative of the established pattern; supra-pubic catheterization may eliminate this problem and is routinely used by some spinal injury centres.
- Symptomatic urinary tract infections alter urodynamic results and should be treated before urodynamic evaluation. Asymptomatic bacteriuria is common and predisposes patients to bacteraemia; it is recommended to use antibiotics 1 hour before the study if necessary.
- Video urodynamics provides the 'gold standard' evaluation of patients who have neurogenic bladder dysfunction. It has the advantage of pressure/flow cystometry while allowing simultaneous anatomical visualization of the bladder and urethra, thus providing information about bladder size and shape, the presence of vesico-ureteric reflux, the competency of the bladder neck and the site of bladder outflow obstruction. Video urodynamics reduces the importance of simultaneous electromyography for diagnosing DSD.

PRACTICAL POINTS IN PERFORMING PRESSURE/FLOW CYSTOMETRY

Performing urodynamics in patients who have neurogenic bladder dysfunction can be challenging and technical modifications may be necessary to obtain the maximum amount of information. Specific issues include:

- Paralysed patients are unable to stand and are best studied in the supine oblique position to obtain maximal visualization of the bladder neck and urethra.
- Voided urine can be transferred from the patient to the flowmeter using a length of guttering, which is fixed to the penis and thigh with tape.
- Sudden bursts of leg or abdominal spasms are not uncommon and may precede detrusor contractions or result in loss of the recording catheters.
- Rectal impaction can theoretically alter vesico-ureteric function during urodynamic evaluation, and rectal evacuation before the study is therefore advised. If suppositories or rectal solutions are used, urodynamics should be delayed until there is a bowel action. Rectal catheterization commonly stimulates bowel evacuation in patients who have a spinal cord injury.
- Trans-urethral catheterization may be difficult in patients who have suprasacral cord lesions because of sphincter spasm.
- Autonomic dysreflexia is a specific risk in this population (see below).

Detrusor leak point pressure

In neurogenic patients who have a high filling pressure the upper tracts have an increased risk of being damaged if there is a subtracted detrusor pressure of more than 30–40 cm H_2O documented during filling cystometry. It is important to realize that neurogenic patients can have dangerously high DLLPs even though they have stress urinary incontinence and low abdominal leak point pressures (ALPP) secondary to intrinsic sphincter deficiency (see Chapter 4).

Autonomic dysreflexia

Autonomic dysreflexia is the exaggerated sympathetic output that occurs in response to a noxious autonomic stimulus below the level of injury in patients who have spinal cord injuries above T6. This manifests as hypertension associated with bradycardia, headache, profuse sweating and flushing above the level of the injury. Spontaneous bladder overdistension or high detrusor pressures may precipitate episodes of autonomic dysreflexia, and may be due to a blocked catheter, inadequate drainage, bladder stones or UTI. Similarly, pressure/flow cystometry may also precipitate autonomic dysreflexia during filling or in relation to DSD and should be prevented by slow filling rates and the maintenance of low volumes and detrusor pressures. Autonomic dysreflexia is a life threatening event and must be treated immediately. All units performing urodynamics on spinal cord injured patients should have a protocol in place for the emergency treatment of the condition.

If autonomic dysreflexia occurs during pressure/flow urodynamics:

- Stop filling and empty the bladder as soon as possible with a large urethral catheter.
- Sit patient up/raise the head.
- Measure the blood pressure.
- Administer sublingual nifedipine 10 mg to lower the blood pressure rapidly.
- Continue treatment and monitoring as per local guidelines.

ELECTROMYOGRAPHY

Electromyography (see Chapter 3) is the study of the bio-electric potentials generated by depolarization of skeletal muscle. The primary value of EMG is for identifying neuropathy. The functional unit in EMG is the motor unit, which is composed of:

- a varying number of muscle fibres supplied by the same motor neurone
- the axon of the motor neurone.

An excitatory impulse in the motor neurone causes each of its muscle fibres to contract and the sum of this activity is called the motor unit action potential (MUAP). The waveform of the MUAP is generally biphasic or triphasic and may be detected by electrodes and displayed on an oscilloscope screen, strip chart or on a urodynamic monitor if performed synchronously with pressure/flow cystometry.

Individually recorded on an oscilloscope, the MUAP has its own amplitude, duration and firing frequency. When a motor neurone is damaged the muscle fibres that have lost their nerve supply become re-innervated by adjacent healthy nerve fibres resulting in fewer but larger motor units. This results in MUAPs of larger amplitude and increased complexity (polyphasic) and duration. These changes in EMG may be used to infer the presence of neurological disease.

170

Types of electrode

Surface electrodes

Surface electrodes (skin, anal plug and catheter) record total electrical output from the muscles of the pelvic floor and are the standard electrodes used in clinical practice. They cannot record individual MUAPs, but allow assessment of overall muscle behaviour. Surface electrodes should be applied to an area as close to the muscle under investigation as possible. They can be difficult to secure and provide less reproducible results than needle electrodes.

Needle electrodes

Individual MUAPs may be detected by needle electrodes placed directly into or near the muscle to be studied. Most commonly the needle is placed directly into the peri-urethral sphincter. A variety of different types of needle electrodes exist including concentric, bipolar, monopolar and single fibre. They permit a more precise recording of EMG activity and analysis of individual MUAPs than surface electrodes. The technique is, however, user dependent and requires considerable expertise; it is also uncomfortable for patients. Its use is therefore generally limited to research and highly specialized centres.

Recording site

EMGs are commonly recorded from three muscles:
1. The external anal sphincter.
2. The levator ani.
3. The striated urethral sphincter.

The easiest muscle to use is the external anal sphincter because placement is simple and dislodgement is less common. In most patients the EMG recorded from the three sites is similar, but in some neurological disorders, particularly demyelinating disease and partial cauda equina lesions, there may be significant differences between the recordings. It is therefore recommended by many to always record from the peri-urethral musculature.

Interpretation

Volitional control of the urinary sphincter is demonstrated by an increase and decrease in EMG activity associated with active contraction and relaxation of the pelvic floor musculature respectively.

During filling there is a normal progressive increase in EMG activity referred to as recruitment. Just prior to voiding the urethral musculature should relax and electrical silence during EMG monitoring is seen

(Appendix 3, example trace 1). This relaxation should persist throughout the detrusor contraction.

Abnormal persistent EMG activity during voiding can be due to:

- the fact that complete electrical silence does not always occur
- straining artefact
- detrusor–sphincter dyssynergia (DSD)
- pelvic floor dyssynergia. (Appendix 3, example trace 5)

In contrast, pseudodyssynergia is the normal voluntary contraction of the external sphincter and pelvic floor muscles in response to an involuntory detrusor contraction (in the filling phase of the study) in an attempt to prevent urgency incontinence.

True DSD occurs only in patients who have neurological disorders. Several patterns of DSD have been described on EMG:

- A crescendo increase in EMG activity that reaches a peak at the peak of the detrusor contraction.
- Alternating contraction and relaxation (clonic EMG activity) of the sphincter musculature during the detrusor contraction (Appendix 3, example trace 4).
- Sustained sphincter contraction throughout the period of the contraction (failure of relaxation).

OTHER SPECIALIZED NEUROPHYSIOLOGICAL STUDIES

Nerve conduction studies

These are performed by stimulating a peripheral nerve and monitoring the time for a response to occur in its innervated muscle. The time until the first measurable muscle response is termed the motor latency. These studies test the integrity of nerve pathways, demonstrating prolonged latencies when there is injury to the nerve with associated demyelination. The most commonly tested latency used to assess neuropathic bladder dysfunction is the bulbocavernosus reflex.

Nerve conduction studies have been found to be beneficial in diagnosing neurological disease, but require elaborate instrumentation and expert interpretation.

Evoked responses

Evoked responses are potential changes in neural tissue resulting from distant stimulation, usually electrical. They are used to test the integrity of peripheral, spinal and central nervous pathways. As with nerve conduction studies, their usage is confined to specialized neurophysiology centres.

Bethanechol supersensitivity test

When an organ is deprived of its nerve supply it will develop hypersensitivity to its own neurotransmitter (Cannon's law of denervation). The bethanechol supersensitivity test is based on this theory; during the test 2.5 mg of bethanechol chloride, an acetylcholine like agent, is administered subcutaneously following an initial pressure/flow study. During a repeat pressure/flow study a rise in detrusor pressure of more than 15 cm H_2O compared to the first study at 100 ml filling is a positive result and implies that the detrusor is denervated. A negative result suggests that the detrusor failure is due to a non-neurological cause.

False negative and false positive results are common and bethanechol is contraindicated for patients who have cardiac disease, hypertension, asthma, peptic ulcer or bladder outlet obstruction. Use of this technique remains contentious.

Ice water test

Cold temperature provokes the bladder and increases detrusor activity. The ice water test is performed by instilling 90 ml of sterile ice-cold water (4°C) into an empty bladder through a 16 Fr catheter without filling the catheter balloon. The test is positive if the catheter is ejected together with a significant amount of water within 1 min of installation (in the absence of straining). A positive result implies that the patient has NDO and may be of some use in diagnosing the cause of incontinence in patients with spinal cord injury (Figure 9.2).

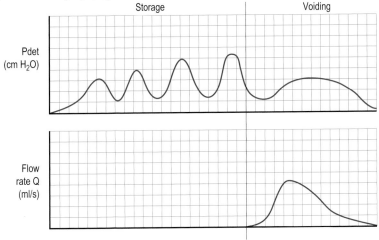

Figure 9.2 *Urodynamic trace*, showing neurogenic detrusor overactivity (NDO) associated with an incompetent urethral mechanism. Note the relatively low voiding pressure and 'normal' flow rate.

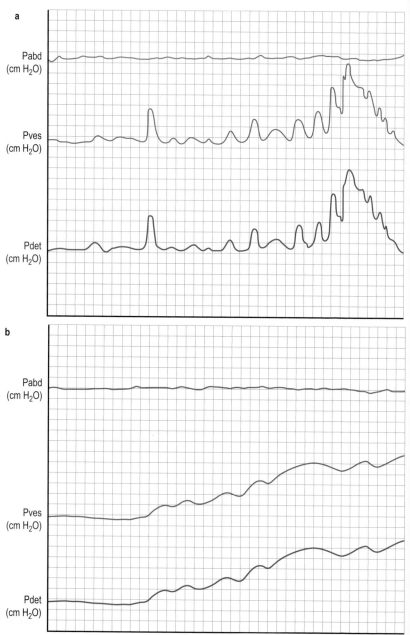

Figure 9.3 **(a) and (b) Patterns of detrusor overactivity frequently seen in neurogenic dysfunction.** (a) *Shows repetitive phasic detrusor contractions with a crescendo and stepping pattern as the bladder volume increases.* (b) *Shows a stepping pattern with consecutive detrusor contractions. It is probable that there is also an underlying decrease in bladder compliance, with the detrusor contractions 'superimposed' upon this.*

NEUROGENIC BLADDER DYSFUNCTION: PRACTICAL POINTS

- Detrusor–sphincter dyssynergia is a pathognomonic feature of suprasacral spinal cord neurogenic bladder dysfunction.
- A number of cystometric patterns are commonly seen in patients with neurogenic bladder:
  - Loss of bladder compliance
  - High pressure detrusor overactivity, often repetitive in a phasic 'systolic' pattern (Figure 9.3a)
  - Detrusor overactivity in a 'stepping pattern' (consecutive detrusor contractions probably superimposed on loss of compliance) (Figure 9.3b).
- Patients with neurogenic bladder may demonstrate a hypo-sensitive bladder or absent bladder sensation.
- Neurogenic patients may not be able to generate a voluntary detrusor contraction.
- Video urodynamics may demonstrate a number of abnormalities:
  - Bladder trabeculation and/or diverticula; or a 'Christmas tree'-shaped bladder
  - Vesico-ureteral reflux
  - Decompensated bladder neck and/or prostatic urethra
  - Bladder neck and/or distal sphincter dyssynergia.

CHAPTER 10

Paediatric urodynamics

INTRODUCTION

Lower urinary tract dysfunction is common in children from both non-neurogenic and neurogenic causes. Most cases are well-recognized functional voiding disorders or have an underlying abnormality such as bladder outlet obstruction, and diagnosis does not depend upon the use of urodynamics. As a general rule, urodynamics is not routinely required in the evaluation of non-neurogenic paediatric voiding dysfunction, since in most cases adequate diagnosis and treatment can be based upon a thorough history and physical examination with appropriate use of endoscopy and radiography. However, urodynamic studies are important investigations in the evaluation and treatment of children with neurogenic bladder dysfunction, commonly due to spinal abnormalities.

Paediatric urodynamics is a highly specialized field and should only be performed in centres with the necessary equipment and expertise.

PAEDIATRIC LOWER URINARY TRACT DYSFUNCTION

As in adults, lower urinary tract dysfunction in children can be categorized as either storage or voiding. These include:

- Storage
  - ○ Incontinence
    - ■ urgency incontinence (most frequent)
    - ■ overflow incontinence
    - ■ other causes of incontinence
  - ○ Nocturnal enuresis.
- Voiding
  - ○ Functional obstruction
  - ○ Mechanical obstruction.

Nocturnal enuresis is 'bedwetting' after the age of 5 years, with no other urinary tract dysfunction. Urodynamic studies are generally not required in the assessment of nocturnal enuresis. Incontinence may be due to a number of causes and a urodynamic study may be helpful in determining the cause and planning the management. Mechanical obstruction in boys may be due to urethral valves, phimosis or meatal stenosis; in girls it may be due to urethral stenosis. Functional obstruction is due to detrusor sphincter dyssynergia (DSD) secondary to a neurological abnormality or secondary to poor relaxation of the pelvic floor and urethral sphincter mechanism.

HISTORY AND EXAMINATION

Most non-neurogenic childhood urinary tract dysfunction do not require urodynamics, therefore a detailed history and physical examination is required to:
- characterize the bladder dysfunction
- look for underlying organic disease
- identify common functional voiding syndromes.

A detailed voiding history is essential and should include:
- age and results of toilet training
- occurrence of primary or secondary enuresis
- specific pattern of wetting, such as stress incontinence, continual dripping or urge incontinence
- manoeuvres used to prevent wetting such as squatting, leg crossing, dancing or 'Vincent's curtsy' (see below)
- frequency of daytime and night-time micturition.

Physical examination should include:
- inspection of the genitalia
- palpation of the lumbosacral spine to detect vertebral defects or sacral agenesis
- examination of the skin overlying the spine for hairy patches, dimples or bumps that might indicate occult spinal abnormalities
- inspection of the lower extremities for subtle neuropathy-related bony abnormalities
- a careful neurological examination.

Investigations should include:
- urinalysis
- post-void residual estimation.

Functional disorders

Functional disorders often resolve spontaneously and usually urodynamic studies add little to the diagnosis and treatment of these children and should be reserved for selected cases. A common pattern is seen in 4 to 7-year-olds; symptoms commonly include frequency and urgency incontinence, yet bladder signals appear to be ignored during play activities. Girls may display the 'Vincent's curtsy' sign where the heel is pressed into the perineum to prevent incontinence secondary to detrusor contractions. Most cases resolve spontaneously, but a number may require a period of anticholinergic medication to alleviate the symptoms.

INDICATIONS FOR URODYNAMICS

Indications for urodynamic investigations in children include:
- Suspected neurogenic dysfunction such as DSD.
- Voiding dysfunction associated with significant bladder hypertrophy, vesico-ureteric reflux or upper urinary tract damage.
- Daytime incontinence that is troublesome for the child, refractory to conservative therapy and is not typical of common functional voiding disorders.
- Symptomatic patients suspected of having occult neuropathy.
- Persistent nocturnal enuresis and recurrent urinary tract infections in some children (rare).

URODYNAMIC INVESTIGATIONS

All urodynamic investigations in children require time, patience and, above all, experienced interpretation.

Uroflowmetry

In general the usefulness of uroflowmetry in the evaluation of paediatric voiding dysfunction is limited because flow rates vary with age, sex and volume voided, preventing the establishment of standard values. The child must be old enough to follow instructions and void in his or her usual fashion; often a normal pattern associated with efficient bladder emptying may be sufficient, making further urodynamic testing unnecessary. Measurement of the post-void residual urine volume with a bladder scanner remains an important part of the clinical evaluation.

Electromyography

Electromyography of the striated muscles of the pelvic floor is necessary to assess the synergy between the bladder and urethral sphincter mechanisms during voiding. Uroflowmetry with simultaneous EMG is frequently performed in children and may help differentiate DSD from abdominal straining during voiding. The EMG electrodes can be placed on the pelvic floor or on the abdominal muscles. Increased EMG activity secondary to straining is common in children and must be differentiated from true detrusor–sphincter dyssynergia, which is diagnostic of neurogenic bladder dysfunction.

EMG is also usually performed concurrently with cystometry (see below). Surface patch electrodes are used in most cases, but fine needle electrodes placed directly into the peri-urethral striated sphincter are recommended to diagnose neuropathy; however, this is not normally feasible in children.

Cystometry

Filling using 5–8 F urethral catheters or feeding tubes is recommended. Filling can be performed transurethrally or in select cases using lines that have been suprapubically inserted under anaesthesia. The suprapubic line should have been in at least 6 hours, although a much longer period prior to performing the study is preferable.

The rectal catheter and EMG surface electrodes can be placed immediately before starting the investigation. If the rectal catheter is not well tolerated, abdominal wall EMG may be used to detect abdominal wall muscle activity, giving an indirect measure of abdominal pressure.

Infusion rates depend upon the cystometric capacity, which is dependent on age. Adults are filled at a rate of approximately 10% of the bladder capacity (i.e. 50 ml/min for a 500 ml capacity bladder). Children should be filled at the same ratio (10–25 ml/min); however in neurogenic dysfunction the rate should be lowered even further. Bladder capacity in children can be calculated from the following formula:

$$\text{Age (years)} \times 30 + 30 = \text{bladder capacity (ml)}$$

The child can be filled in a supine or sitting position and should be encouraged to void in a position and fashion that is as normal as possible. Ideally children should be fully awake during cystometry, but in some cases mild sedation is required to obtain useful information.

Video urodynamics

Video urodynamics provides a more comprehensive evaluation especially in patients who have neurogenic bladder dysfunction, bladder outlet obstruction and incontinence.

Detrusor–sphincter dyssynergia can be diagnosed during fluoroscopy without direct measurement of EMG activity, eliminating the need for potentially bothersome electrodes.

URODYNAMICS IN PRACTICE: PAEDIATRIC PATIENTS

- An urodynamic investigation is only useful if it can be performed without undue anxiety; patient co-operation allowing reproduction of the normal voiding pattern is of utmost importance to obtain useful clinical information.
- A pleasant, cheerful testing environment and staff, and the presence of a family member will help reduce fear and anxiety.
- Common helpful distracters include movies, television, games, toys and favourite treats.

INTERPRETATION

Because of the great variability in the development of urinary control in young children, extreme caution is needed in interpreting their urodynamics and in diagnosing disorders of lower urinary tract function. Urodynamics must therefore not be undertaken lightly in this group and must be interpreted with care.

It is likely that all children transiently display abnormalities in bladder and sphincter function when making the transition from infantile to adult patterns of urinary control. Provided that these are not sustained, they do not appear to be pathological or to carry any long term consequences.

As with adult pressure/flow studies, cystometry provides useful information about bladder capacity, sensation, compliance and detrusor/urethral function. The maximum cystometric capacity is often lower than the calculated anatomical capacity and depends upon the child's ability to suppress voiding.

An estimation of bladder sensitivity (hyper-sensitive, hypo-sensitive or normal) can be made during filling. Filling is usually limited by:

- a sensation of bladder fullness or even pain
- urinary incontinence secondary to detrusor overactivity or poor detrusor compliance
- uncontrollable spontaneous voiding.

Detrusor overactivity – May or may not represent a clinically significant abnormality, depending upon the child's age and voluntary response to the overactivity. Overactive contractions are considered to be normal in young immature bladders until central inhibitory pathways develop fully, even in the face of a strong desire to void. This maturation usually occurs by 4 years of age, and often much earlier. Prior to maturation voiding is involuntary and usually to completion, as a result of a well-sustained detrusor contraction accompanied by synergic relaxation of the urethral sphincter mechanism.

181

Dysfunctional voiding – Voluntary contraction of the external sphincter in an attempt to prevent incontinence is common in the early development of normal urinary control. This results in an obstruction to flow with high intra-vesical pressure. In some children, this 'voluntary dyssynergia' can remain, resulting in long term voiding dysfunction. Renal damage can result in the most severe of cases. This pattern of dysfunctional voiding is known as Hinman's syndrome and was also previously termed 'non-neuropathic neuropathic bladder'.

DSD – Voluntary contraction of the external sphincter to prevent leakage during involuntary detrusor contractions is commonly misinterpreted as DSD in patients who do not have neuropathy. This is an appropriate patient response in an attempt to maintain continence and can be referred to as 'pseudodyssynergia'. To make the important distinction between DSD and pseudodyssynergia, the patient should be asked to void voluntarily. During DSD continued EMG activity in the external sphincter will occur, whereas in pseudodyssynergia the EMG activity should become silent.

Compliance – Reduced bladder compliance is commonly found in children who have neurogenic bladder dysfunction. The pre-micturition pressure is normally below 10 cm H_2O. Children who have myelomeningocoele and reduced bladder compliance with a detrusor leak point pressure of over 40 cm H_2O are at risk of renal damage as a result of the high detrusor pressure.

Scheme for performing a pressure/flow study

In this appendix a scheme for performing a pressure/flow study is summarized. It is good practice to perform urodynamics in a standard routine to ensure that all the possible data are obtained. However, each individual study should be modified to ensure that the urodynamic question and other relevant data are fully obtained without undue effort being spent obtaining clinically irrelevant data. In addition the scheme should be modified depending on local facilities.

PRIOR TO TEST – PATIENT FACTORS

- Reassess clinical history and the 'urodynamic question'.
- Physical examination if necessary.
- Obtain consent for procedure.
- Assess voiding diary to determine bladder capacity at which to stop filling (if not previously done).
- Perform initial free uroflowmetry for comparison and quality control (if not previously done).
- Exclude UTI (urinalysis).
- Consider if prophylactic antibiotics are necessary.

PRIOR TO TEST – EQUIPMENT FACTORS AND SETUP

- Ensure equipment is calibrated, setup correctly and functioning.
- Insert intra-vesical measuring and filling lines with patient in supine position using an aseptic technique (and lidocaine gel in men).
- Insert intra-abdominal measuring line with patient in left lateral position; ensure slit is cut in rectal balloon.
- Drain bladder to assess the initial residual urine or fill on top of the initial residual and calculate initial residual later.
- Connect catheters to transducers/recording equipment and filling pump.
- Flush fluid lines, ensure all air bubbles from both the tubing and transducer chambers have been excluded.

- Zero to atmospheric pressure (perform this prior to catheter insertion if using microtip catheters).
- Set reference height to level of pubic symphysis.
- Ensure resting values are within the expected range.
- Ensure no dampening is present.

STARTING THE TEST

- Begin recording.
- Perform a quality control cough and repeat every 1 minute (and before and after any events).
- Start filling at the desired rate.
- Adjust patient position, standing is preferable (many urodynamicists stand the patient when the first sensation of filling occurs).
- Adjust reference height with each change of patient position.
- Maintain constant interaction with the patient.
- Monitor the intra-abdominal, intra-vesical and subtracted detrusor traces throughout the study.

STORAGE PHASE

- Ensure patient is trying to suppress voiding/leakage during the storage phase.
- Record volume of first sensation of filling, first desire to void, strong desire to void.
- Record any episodes of urgency and/or leakage.
- Assess for stress incontinence with intermittent coughs/valsalva (in oblique position if using video screening, or if screening is not available with the patient lying flat with legs abducted or standing with legs slightly apart).
- Perform leak point pressure measurements if desired.
- Determine bladder compliance.
- Record episodes of detrusor overactivity (DO) including volume at which they occur, maximum rise in pressure and any associated urgency/leakage.
- Record the maximum cystometric capacity (MCC).
- Perform provocation tests at MCC if DO not previously detected.
- Use screening (if performing video urodynamics) to assess the bladder outline, volume, vesico-ureteric reflux, diverticula, trabeculations, opening of bladder neck, bladder neck descent, bladder neck hypermobility, leakage.
- Characterize the bladder and urethral function during the storage phase.

VOIDING PHASE

- Ensure patient coughs prior to voiding.
- Record the pre-micturition pressure.
- Allow patient to void.
- Use screening to outline the urethra and determine site of any obstruction, completeness of emptying and presence of any vesico-ureteric reflux.
- Perform stop test if desired.
- On completion of voiding ensure patient coughs again.
- Adjust flow trace for flow rate delay.
- Record voiding parameters including maximum detrusor pressure, maximum flow rate, detrusor pressure at maximum flow rate, volume voided.
- Assess residual urine (and calculate initial residual if necessary).
- Assess for BOO using ICS nomogram.
- Characterize the bladder and urethral function during the voiding phase.
- Consider urethral pressure profilometry if felt appropriate.

AT THE END OF STUDY

- Determine whether study needs repeating.
- Complete study pro-forma if used.
- Discuss findings with patient.
- Write study report and plan for further investigation/management.
- Ensure data is printed and suitably archived electronically.

Normal urodynamic values

Some pertinent normal urodynamic values are listed in this appendix. These serve only as a guide and all urodynamic findings should be interpreted with knowledge of the history, physical examination, investigation results and findings from other urodynamic investigations. No urodynamic findings should be considered in isolation as this will invariably lead to the incorrect interpretation of the results.

PAD TESTING

With the 1-hour International Continence Society pad test, the upper limit (99% confidence limit) has been found to be 1.4 g/hour. (Although it may be as high as 2.1 g/hour in women who consider themselves continent.)

UROFLOWMETRY

Men under 40 years = Q_{max} > 25 ml/s.
Men over 60 years = Q_{max} > 15 ml/s.
Females   = Q_{max} > 30–35 ml/s.

PRESSURE/FLOW STUDIES

Storage

Maximum cystometric capacity (MCC) = 350–600 ml.
Volume at first sensation   = approx 50% of the MCC.
Volume at normal desire   = approx 75% of the MCC.
Volume at strong desire   = approx 90% of the MCC.
Normal compliance   = >30 ml/cm H_2O.

Voiding

Maximum detrusor pressure	$= 25\text{–}60$ cm H_2O.
$P_{det}@Q_{max}$ in men	$= 40\text{–}60$ cm H_2O.
$P_{det}@Q_{max}$ in females	$= 20\text{–}40$ cm H_2O.
Post-void residual	$= {<}25$ ml.

Bladder outlet obstruction index (BOOI)	$= {>}20$ obstructed.
BOOI	$= 20\text{–}40$ equivocal.
BOOI	$= {<}20$ unobstructed.

Leak point pressures and urethral pressure profilometry (UPP)

(These values are not universally accepted and remain an area of dispute.)

- Abdominal leak point pressure (ALPP) >100 cm H_2O: suggests urethral hypermobility.
- ALPP <60 cm H_2O: suggests intrinsic sphincter deficiency (ISD).
- Detrusor leak point pressure (DLPP) >40 cm H_2O: suggests upper tract deterioration likely.
- Maximum urethral closure pressure <20 cm H_2O: suggests intrinsic sphincter deficiency (ISD).

Example traces

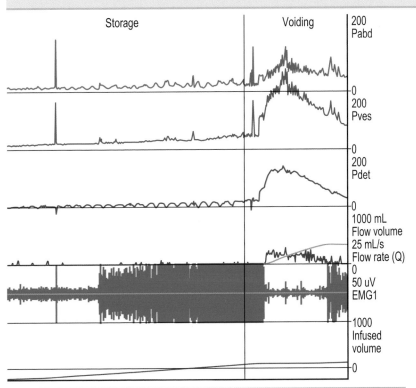

	Storage phase	Voiding phase
Detrusor function	Normal, although rectal contractions give the misleading appearance of phasic detrusor overactivity	Overactive (high pressure)
Urethral/bladder outlet function	Normal; increased EMG activity due to rectal contractions and recruitment (See chapter 9)	Prolonged, low flow (obstructive): appropriate decrease in EMG activity with voiding
Quality	Dampening of intra-vesical line, rectal contractions throughout, artefactual movements to flowmeter during storage phase	
Diagnosis	Bladder outlet obstruction	

Table A3.1

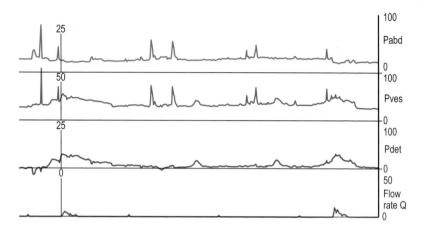

	Storage phase	Voiding phase
Detrusor function	Detrusor overactivity following coughing	Not shown
Urethral/bladder outlet function	Urinary incontinence due to detrusor overactivity	Not shown
Quality	Acceptable	
Diagnosis	Cough induced detrusor overactivity with incontinence	

Table A3.2

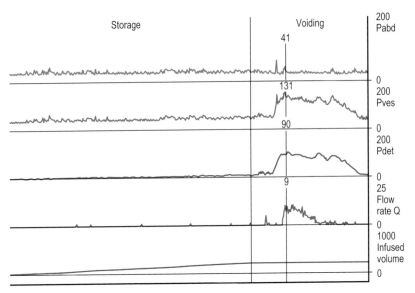

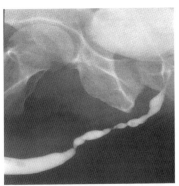

	Storage phase	Voiding phase
Detrusor function	Normal	High pressure (overactive)
Urethra/bladder outlet function	Normal	Low flow rate (<9 ml/s)
Quality	Subtraction appears acceptable, although no quality control coughs	
Diagnosis	BOO and superimposed screening image shows a urethral stricture	

Table A3.3

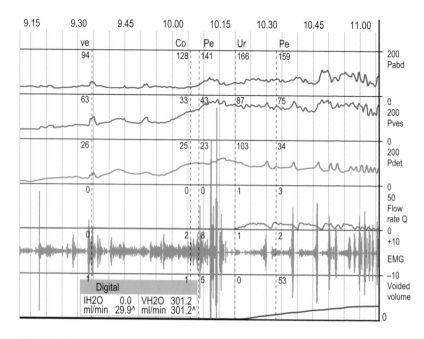

	Storage phase	Voiding phase
Detrusor function	Overactive; recurrent contractions with 'stepping' pattern	High pressure involuntary void (overactive)
Urethral/bladder outlet function	Competent	Intermittent flow with corresponding rises in detrusor pressure. EMG shows intermittent sphincter activity
Quality	No quality control coughs but subtraction appears acceptable	
Diagnosis	Neurogenic detrusor overactivity and DSD	

Table A3.4

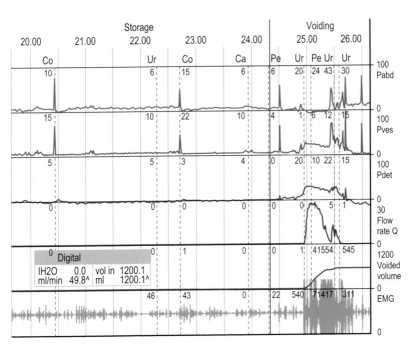

First sensation	925 ml infused volume
MCC	1182 ml infused volume
Q_{max}	29 ml/s
pDet @ Q_{max}	24 cm H_2O
Voided volume	585 ml

	Storage phase	Voiding phase
Detrusor function	Hypo-sensitive with late first sensation at 925 ml filling and large cystometric capacity of 1182 ml	Low pressure (P_{det}@ Q_{max} = 24 cm H_2O)
Urethra/bladder outlet function	Competent	Normal peak flow (29 ml/s), incomplete emptying (voided only 585 ml); increased EMG activity during voiding
Quality	Acceptable	
Diagnosis	Hypo-sensitive, large capacity bladder Possibly low detrusor pressure secondary to overdistension or developing poor detrusor contractility (detrusor failure) Increased EMG activity compatible with DSD or pelvic floor dyssynergia	

Table A3.5

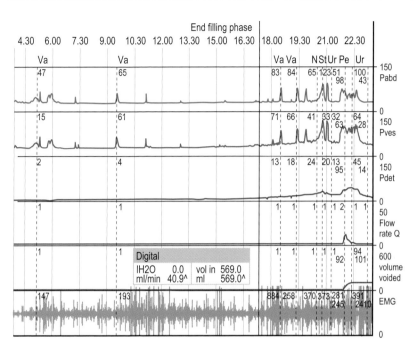

	Storage phase	Voiding phase
Detrusor function	Normal	Low pressure void associated with abdominal straining
Urethral/bladder outlet function	Competent	Low flow rate with incomplete emptying; increased EMG activity compatible with abdominal straining
Quality	Acceptable	
Diagnosis	Poor detrusor contractility (detrusor failure)	

Table A3.6

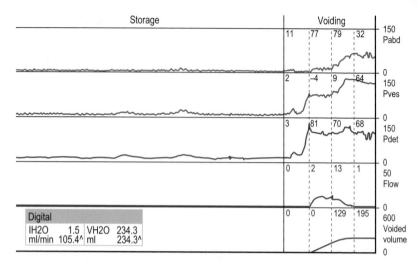

	Storage phase	Voiding phase
Detrusor function	Overactive	High pressure, although the subtraction does not appear to be accurate
Urethral/bladder outlet function	Competent	Low flow rate with additional abdominal straining
Quality	Quality control coughs not present, poor subtraction during voiding phase	
Diagnosis	Bladder outlet obstruction and detrusor overactivity	

Table A3.7

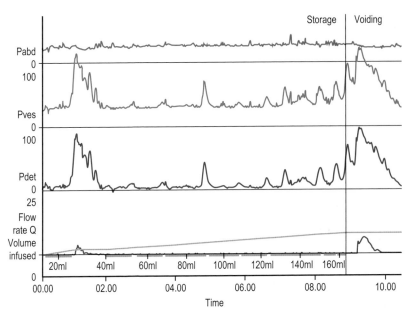

	Storage phase	Voiding phase
Detrusor function	Phasic detrusor overactivity	High pressure
Urethral/bladder outlet function	Leakage associated with detrusor overactivity	Low flow rate
Quality	Few quality control coughs, intra-abdominal line dampening	
Diagnosis	Gross detrusor overactivity with incontinence, unable to interpret voiding phase as void is initiated during a terminal contraction; the appearance of obstruction in this case may be due to the abnormally high pressures present at the start of voiding. Patient should have the voiding phase repeated to accurately define the voiding function	

Table A3.8

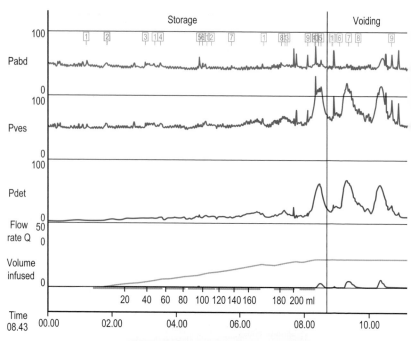

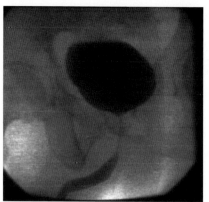

	Storage phase	Voiding phase
Detrusor function	Overactive	High pressure
Urethral/bladder outlet function	Competent	Intermittent low flow rate with incomplete emptying and prostatic obstruction visible on screening image
Quality	Dampening in abdominal line. No coughs.	
Diagnosis	Detrusor overactivity and BOO secondary to prostatic obstruction	

Table A3.9

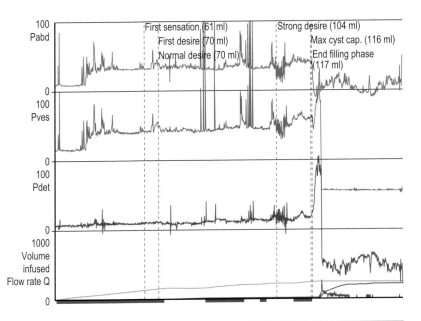

	Storage phase	Voiding phase
Detrusor function	Overactive and oversensitive with first sensation at 61 ml filling and MCC at 116 ml filling. Possible overactivity but poor subtraction makes identification difficult.	Uninterpretable. Due to loss of urethral catheter.
Urethral/bladder outlet function	Competent	Poor flow with some abdominal straining
Quality	Dampening in abdominal line throughout study. Intra-vesical catheter voided out at the beginning of voiding phase.	
Diagnosis	Oversensitivity and possible detrusor overactivity; study needs repeating to determine detrusor function during voiding and storage phases with better quality control.	

Table A3.10

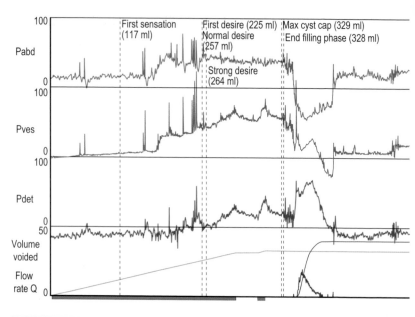

	Storage phase	Voiding phase
Detrusor function	Overactive	Normal pressure (P_{det} falsely elevated at end of filling due to drop in rectal pressue; voiding pressure appears normal based on P_{ves})
Urethral/bladder outlet function	Competent	Normal flow pattern, slightly low Q_{max}. Need to perform free uroflowmetry to determine Q_{max} without an in situ catheter
Quality	High P_{abd} at baseline causing a negative detrusor pressure. Dampening of intra-abdominal line throughout study. Immediately prior to voiding patient changed position to sitting with no alteration in reference height. Poor quality assessment	
Diagnosis	Detrusor overactivity	

Table A3.11

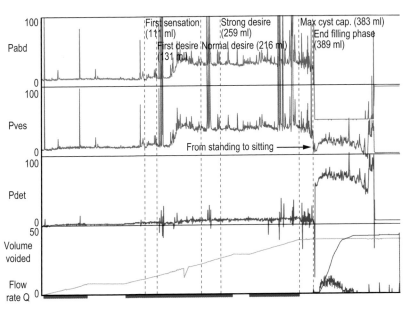

	Storage phase	Voiding phase
Detrusor function	Normal	Uninterpretable due to loss of intra-abdominal line although possibly poor detrusor contractility
Urethral/bladder outlet function	Competent	Poor flow
Quality	Intra-abdominal catheter passed out at the beginning of voiding	
Diagnosis	Study needs repeating to determine subtracted detrusor function during voiding once intra-abdominal line is replaced.	

Table A3.12

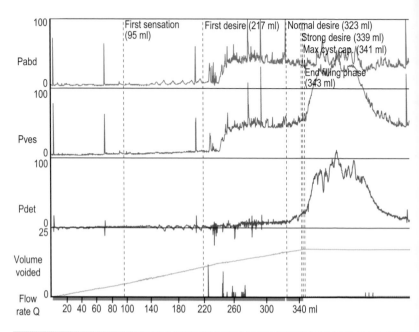

	Storage phase	Voiding phase
Detrusor function	Rectal contractions only	Overactive (high pressure)
Urethral/bladder outlet function	Competent (flow readings are artefacts)	Negligible flow despite additional abdominal straining
Quality	Impaired subtraction throughout study noticeable on quality control coughs	
Diagnosis	High pressure BOO	

Table A3.13

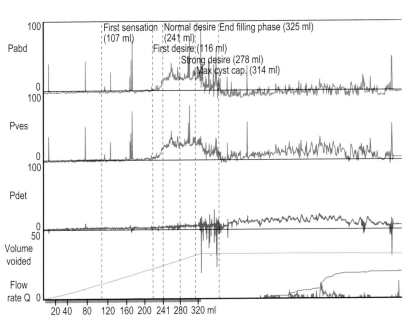

	Storage phase	Voiding phase
Detrusor function	Early bladder sensations suggesting some oversensitivity	Severely hypo-contractile, with a prolonged time before commencing any voiding. Intermittent voiding with a negligible amount passed
Urethra/bladder outlet function	Competent	Low pressure, low flow voiding despite abdominal straining
Quality	Slight dampening in abdominal line throughout study. Intra-abdominal pressure is artefactually negative during parts of the study leading to artefactual rise in detrusor pressure	
Diagnosis	Detrusor failure (possibly some oversensitivity)	

Table A3.14

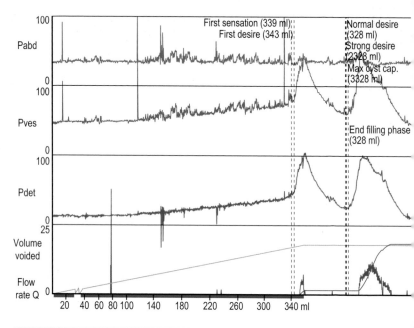

	Storage phase	Voiding phase
Detrusor function	Poor detrusor compliance Overactive with associated incontinence	No voluntary void, voided off an overactive contraction
Urethral/bladder outlet function	Leakage associated with DO	No voluntary void
Quality	Occasional dampening in intra-abdominal line	
Diagnosis	Detrusor overactivity and poor bladder compliance	

Table A3.15

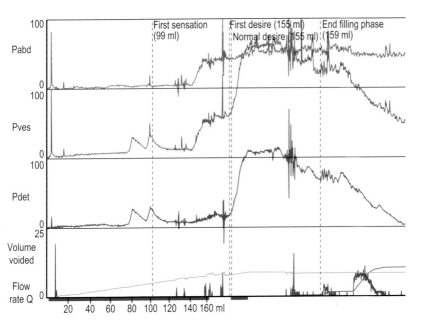

Storage phase labels: First sensation (99 ml); First desire (155 ml); Normal desire (155 ml); End filling phase (159 ml)

Traces: Pabd, Pves, Pdet, Volume voided, Flow rate Q

x-axis: 20 40 60 80 100 120 140 160 ml

	Storage phase	Voiding phase
Detrusor function	Overactive, with several small involuntary contractions followed by a large terminal contraction Early sensations suggesting some oversensitivity	Voided during a terminal contraction
Urethral/bladder outlet function	Incompetent on coughing	Normal flow pattern
Quality	Dampening in abdominal line throughout study	
Diagnosis	Mixed incontinence, with some degree of oversensitivity; cannot interpret voiding phase as voided off an overactive contraction	

Table A3.16

Bibliography

FURTHER READING

It is clear that urodynamic evaluation is essential for the accurate investigation of patients who have lower urinary tract symptoms. As only a brief summary of this subject can be provided here, comprehensive reviews should be consulted for more detailed information:

Abrams P 2006 Urodynamics, 3rd edn. London: Springer.

Abrams P, Cardozo L, Khoury S, Wein A 2005 Incontinence. Paris: Health Publications Ltd.

These are the reports from the 3rd International Consultation on Incontinence. ISBN 0-9546956-2-3. They are also available on the ICS website (www.icsoffice.org)

Mundy AR, Stephenson TP, Wein AJ, eds 1994 Urodynamics – Principles, Practice and Application, 2nd edn. Edinburgh: Churchill Livingstone.

Patel U, Rickards D 2005 Imaging and Urodynamics of the Lower Urinary Tract, 1st edn. Oxford: Taylor and Francis.

Wein AJ, Kavoussi LR, Novick AC, Partin AW, Peters CA 2006 Campbell-Walsh Urology, 9th edn. Edinburgh: Elsevier.

ICS DOCUMENTS AND REPORTS

The International Continence Society (ICS) has produced a number of standardization reports and documents regarding lower urinary tract dysfunction and investigation. These have been published widely and are also available on the ICS website (www.icsoffice.org). Recent reports include:

Abrams P, Cardozo L, Fall M, Griffiths D, Rosier P, Ulmsten U et al 2002 The standardisation of terminology of lower urinary tract function: report from the Standardisation Sub-committee of the International Continence Society. Neurourol Urodyn 21: 167–78.

Griffiths D, Hofner K, van Mastrigt R, Rollema HJ, Spangberg A, Gleason D 1997 Standardization of terminology of lower urinary tract function: pressure–flow studies of voiding, urethral resistance, and urethral obstruction. International Continence Society Subcommittee on Standardization of Terminology of Pressure–Flow Studies. Neurourol Urodyn 16: 1–18.

Lose G, Griffiths D, Hosker G, Kulseng-Hanssen S, Perucchini D, Schafer W et al 2002 Standardisation of urethral pressure measurement: report from the Standardisation Sub-Committee of the International Continence Society. Neurourol Urodyn 21: 258–60.

Messelink B, Benson T, Berghmans B, Bo K, Corcos J, Fowler C et al 2005 Standardization of terminology of pelvic floor muscle function and dysfunction: report from the pelvic floor clinical assessment group of the International Continence Society. Neurourol Urodyn 24: 374–80.

Schafer W, Abrams P, Liao L, Mattiasson A, Pesce F, Spangberg A et al 2002 Good urodynamic practices: uroflowmetry, filling cystometry, and pressure–flow studies. Neurourol Urodyn 21: 261–74.

Stohrer M, Goepel M, Kondo A, Kramer G, Madersbacher H, Millard R et al 1999 The standardization of terminology in neurogenic lower urinary tract dysfunction: with suggestions for diagnostic procedures. International Continence Society Standardization Committee. Neurourol Urodyn 18: 139–58.

van Kerrebroeck P, Abrams P, Chaikin D, Donovan J, Fonda D, Jackson S et al 2002 The standardisation of terminology in nocturia: report from the Standardisation Sub-committee of the International Continence Society. Neurourol Urodyn 21: 179–83.

van Mastrigt R, Griffiths DJ 2004 ICS standard for digital exchange of urodynamic study data. Neurourol Urodyn 23: 280–81.

van Waalwijk van Doorn E, Anders K, Khullar V, Kulseng-Hanssen S, Pesce F, Robertson A et al 2000 Standardisation of ambulatory urodynamic monitoring: Report of the Standardisation Sub-Committee of the International Continence Society for Ambulatory Urodynamic Studies. Neurourol Urodyn 19: 113–25.

CLINICAL GUIDELINES

Clinical Guidelines for the assessment and management of lower urinary tract disorders have been produced by a number of organizations including:

- **European Association of Urology (EAU)**: www.uroweb.org
- **American Urological Association (AUA)**: www.auanet.org
- **United Kingdom National Institute for Health and Clinical Excellence (NICE)**: www.nice.org.uk

- **International Consultation on Incontinence (ICI)**: reports available from www.icsoffice.org

- **International Consultation on Urological Diseases (ICUD)**, such as the proceedings of the International consultation on bengin prostatic hyperplasia

Up-to-date guidelines from these and other national and regional bodies should be consulted when assessing and managing patients with lower urinary tract dysfunction.

Index

Q

R

W

Z